Mental Health in Historical Perspective

Series Editors

Covering all historical periods and geographical contexts, the series explores how mental illness has been understood, experienced, diagnosed, treated and contested. It will publish works that engage actively with contemporary debates related to mental health and, as such, will be of interest not only to historians, but also mental health professionals, patients and policy makers. With its focus on mental health, rather than just psychiatry, the series will endeavour to provide more patient-centred histories. Although this has long been an aim of health historians, it has not been realised, and this series aims to change that.

The scope of the series is kept as broad as possible to attract good quality proposals about all aspects of the history of mental health from all periods. The series emphasises interdisciplinary approaches to the field of study, and encourages short titles, longer works, collections, and titles which stretch the boundaries of academic publishing in new ways.

Owen Rees · Kathryn Hurlock · Jason Crowley
Editors

Combat Stress in Pre-modern Europe

palgrave
macmillan

Editors
Owen Rees
Department of History, Politics
and Philosophy
Manchester Metropolitan University
Manchester, UK

Kathryn Hurlock
Department of History, Politics
and Philosophy
Manchester Metropolitan University
Manchester, UK

Jason Crowley
Department of History, Politics
and Philosophy
Manchester Metropolitan University
Manchester, UK

ISSN 2634-6036 ISSN 2634-6044 (electronic)
Mental Health in Historical Perspective
ISBN 978-3-031-09946-5 ISBN 978-3-031-09947-2 (eBook)
https://doi.org/10.1007/978-3-031-09947-2

Cover illustration: insidefoto srl/Alamy Stock Photo

This Palgrave Macmillan imprint is published by the registered company Springer Nature Switzerland AG
The registered company address is: Gewerbestrasse 11, 6330 Cham, Switzerland

A Note on References

A project that brought together such an array of historians covering very different time periods required a little editorial flexibility when it came to the formatting of references. When abbreviations have been used for ancient evidence, they follow the list of abbreviations given in the Oxford Classical Dictionary, 4th edition.

Contents

List of Contributors

Ball Joanne E. University of Liverpool, Liverpool, UK

Christoforou Constantine University of Roehampton, London, UK

Crowley Jason Department of History, Politics and Philosophy, Manchester Metropolitan University, Manchester, UK

Fear Andrew University of Manchester, Manchester, UK

Grosskopf Chelsea University of Iceland, Reykjavík, Iceland

Hurlock Kathryn Department of History, Politics and Philosophy, Manchester Metropolitan University, Manchester, UK

Pells Ismini University of Oxford, Oxford, UK

Proietti Giorgia University of Trento, Trento, Italy

Rees Owen Department of History, Politics and Philosophy, Manchester Metropolitan University, Manchester, UK

Combat Trauma in Pre-modern Europe: An Introduction

Kathryn Hurlock, Owen Rees, and Jason Crowley

Since the genesis of 'shell shock', the pre-modern world has been used to aid our understanding of the psychological and moral injuries incurred during military service. However, the historical study of combat trauma is a contentious topic, not least because of debates over the applicability of modern medical ideas to the conflicts of the past. Despite this problem, research on combat stress in the modern era has regularly drawn upon the past for inspiration and validation, but to date no single volume has effectively scrutinised the universal nature of combat stress and its associated diagnoses. This volume offers cutting-edge research from experts in history, classics, and medical humanities. There are pivotal points of

K. Hurlock (✉) · O. Rees · J. Crowley
Department of History, Politics and Philosophy, Manchester Metropolitan University, Manchester, UK
e-mail: k.hurlock@mmu.ac.uk

O. Rees
e-mail: O.Rees@mmu.ac.uk

J. Crowley
e-mail: J.Crowley@mmu.ac.uk

O. Rees et al. (eds.), *Combat Stress in Pre-modern Europe*, Mental Health in Historical Perspective,
https://doi.org/10.1007/978-3-031-09947-2_1

divergence between papers, offering a dynamic and engaging academic discourse on an important and timely topic. What makes the volume unique is its broad chronological focus, with chapters covering periods from Archaic Greece (sixth and early fifth centuries BCE) to the British Civil Wars of the seventeenth century. This broad chronology is held together through a direct focus on the topic of combat stress, and how it may or may not manifest in different time periods and within different cultural contexts. Topics range from the methodological—such as the issue of retrospective diagnosis, and the applicability of Moral Injury onto the past—to the conventionally historical. The majority of the book focuses on combatants, but there are also chapters examining the impact on women and children, as well as collective trauma for the community.

This volume originated as a small workshop entitled *Combat Stress and the Pre-Modern World* held at Manchester Metropolitan University, UK, in 2018. The purpose of the workshop was not to go over the large body of research that has built up over the past 25 years on the topic of pre-modern combat trauma, but to highlight the new directions that this research was going. It was not about rehashing old arguments but rather looking forward to new questions, new forms of analysis, and possible resolutions. The scholarly focus in this area has situated most of the analysis in classical Greece, so an attempt to bring together scholars from ancient, medieval, and early modern studies was considered critical. Alas, the one area that neither this workshop—nor indeed this volume—could satisfactorily cover was cultural perspectives outside of the European sphere.

From the turn of the millennium, there has been a surge of research that has tried to identify the symptomology of combat stress and post-traumatic stress in the source material, leading to the retrospective diagnosis of such prominent figures as Achilles, Alexander the Great, and Samuel Pepys, to name but a few.[1] The argument that experience is similar enough in the historical past as to be almost a constant has also

[1] Jonathan Shay, *Achilles in Vietnam: Combat Trauma and the Undoing of Character* (New York: Atheneum, 1994); Philip A. Macowiak, 'Post-traumatic Stress Reactions before the Advent of Post-traumatic Stress Disorder: Potential Effects on the Lives and Legacies of Alexander the Great, Captain James Cook, Emily Dickinson, and Florence Nightingale', *Military Medicine* 173, 2008, 1158–63, accessed at https://doi.org/10.7205/milmed.173.12.1158; Alexandra F. Morris, 'Alexander the Great: Head to Head with CTW (Chronic Traumatic Encephalopathy)', *Athens Journal of History* 3, 1983, 225–34, accessed at https://doi.org/10.30958/ajhis.3-3-3; R.J. Daly, 'Samuel Pepys and

been advanced through such influential works as that of Walid Abdul-Hamid and Jamie Hughes.[2] This approach is built on a foundation of universalism. It starts from the belief that humans are innately the same, and while cultures and personalities can change, an integral continuity combines all people in their biology and neurology. As one of the leading proponents of this universalist perspective, ancient historian Lawrence Tritle summarises this view concisely:

> The ability of scientists to trace human DNA to its remote origins by sequencing the DNA of living humans argues for the continuity of human biology—and so the universality of trauma—over the last 150,000 years.[3]

The topics of combat stress and associated injuries are more prevalent in ancient history monographs, but do not offer an academic dialogue; instead, they present a strong argument for the universalist view of combat stress. Key among them is Lawrence Tritle's *Melos to My Lai* which argues strongly for the historicity of Jonathan Shay's more literary analysis of the Homeric epics. He identifies key examples from Classical Greek evidence which have become the lynchpin for the universalist position: Epizelus, the Athenian who went blind at Marathon; Aristodemus, the Spartan who survived the battle of Thermopylae and committed suicide during the battle of Plataea; Clearchus, the Spartan commander of the Ten Thousand; and an extract by the sophist Gorgias which describes the lasting effect of fear in the minds of combatants.[4]

A broader universalist approach can be found within edited volumes on the subject, such as Meineck and Konstan's collection on *Combat Trauma*

Post-traumatic Stress Disorder', *British Journal of Psychiatry* 143, 1983, 64–8, accessed at https://doi.org/10.1192/bjp.143.1.64.

[2] Walid Khalid Abdul-Hamid and Jamie Hacker Hughes, 'Nothing New under the Sun: Post-traumatic Stress Disorders in the Ancient World', *Early Science and Medicine* 19.6, 2014, 549–57, accessed at https://doi.org/10.1163/15733823-00196p02.

[3] Lawrence Tritle, '"Ravished Minds" in the Ancient World', in Peter Meineck and David Konstan (eds), *Combat Trauma and the Ancient Greeks* (New York: Palgrave Macmillan, 2014), pp. 87–104. See also discussion on 'a universal species ethic' in Shay, *Achilles in Vietnam*, p. 208.

[4] L. Tritle, *Melos to My Lai* (London: Routledge, 2000), pp. 61–78; for his analysis of Gorgias, see Lawrence Tritle, 'Gorgias, the Encomium of Helen, and the Trauma of War', *Clio's Psyche* 16.2, 2009, 195–9.

and the Ancient Greeks,[5] and Caston and Weineck's edited volume on *Rethinking War Through the Classics*.[6] Within these, we see excellent pieces of scholarship exploring themes such as trust and betrayal,[7] survivor's guilt,[8] and the presentation of trauma in drama.[9] Indeed, a general acceptance of universalism, with notable caveats,[10] has allowed researchers to focus on the experience of combat and more recently the effects of war on non-combatants, and in society more generally through new areas of analyses such as collective trauma (see Proietti in this volume).[11] It has also inspired some important outreach work such as the Theatre of War Project, founded by Bryan Doerries and Phyllis Kaufman, which uses dramatic readings and performances of historic literature followed by town hall-style discussions to highlight key social issues including war and mental health. In many ways, this is where the concept of ancient PTSD was first proposed, in the revolutionary work of Dr

[5] Peter Meineck and David Konstan (eds), *Combat Trauma and the Ancient Greeks* (New York: Palgrave Macmillan, 2014).

[6] Victor Caston and Silke-Maria Weineck (eds), *Our Ancient Wars: Rethinking War Through the Classics* (Ann Arbor: University of Michigan Press, 2016).

[7] Nancy Sherman, '"He Gave Me His Hand But Took My Bow": Trust and Trustworthiness in the Philoctetes and Our Wars', in Peter Meineck and David Konstan (eds), *Combat Trauma and the Ancient Greeks* (New York: Palgrave Macmillan, 2014), pp. 207–24.

[8] Sharon L. James, 'The Battered Shield: Survivor's Guilt and Family Trauma in Menander's Aspis', in Peter Meineck and David Konstan (eds), *Combat Trauma and the Ancient Greeks* (New York: Palgrave Macmillan, 2014), 237–60.

[9] Peter Meineck, 'Combat Trauma and the Tragic Stage: Ancient Culture and Modern Catharsis?', in Victor Caston and Silke-Maria Weineck (eds), *Our Ancient Wars: Rethinking War Through the Classics* (Ann Arbor: University of Michigan Press, 2016), pp. 184–208.

[10] E.g. S.S. Monoson, 'Socrates in Combat: Trauma and Resilience in Plato's Political Theory', in P. Meineck and D. Konstan (eds), *Combat Trauma and the Ancient Greeks* (New York: Palgrave Macmillan, 2014), pp. 131–62.

[11] Sorkin Rabinowitz, Nancy, 'Women and War in Tragedy', in Peter Meineck and David Konstan (eds), *Combat Trauma and the Ancient Greeks* (New York: Palgrave Macmillan, 2014), pp. 207–25; Kurt Raaflaub, 'Lysistrata and War's Impact on the Home Front', in Victor Caston and Silke-Maria Weineck (eds), *Our Ancient Wars: Rethinking War Through the Classics* (Ann Arbor: University of Michigan Press, 2016), pp. 38–74; Giorgia Proietti, 'Athens as a "Landscape of Trauma": Phrynichus' Sack of Miletus and the Aftermath of the Persian Wars', in Lucia Cecchet, Christopher Degelmann, and Maik Patzelt (eds), *The Ancient War's Impact on the Home Front* (Newcastle-upon-Tyne: Cambridge Scholars, 2019), pp. 79–98.

Jonathan Shay who used the Homeric epics, the *Iliad* and the *Odyssey*, to help his Vietnam veteran clients navigate their own experiences of war and trauma.[12]

This universalist approach has recently been challenged by what is known as the relativist position, giving birth to an important debate about the use of the modern PTSD model as a way to explore pre-modern combat, and post-combat, experiences.[13] Relativist scholars challenge the argument that the experience of warfare is universal or that PTSD can be found across time and space.[14] The strongest assertions of the relativist position comes from anthropologist Allan Young—who argues that PTSD and traumatic memory do not occur before the nineteenth century—and psychiatrist Derek Summerfield—who challenges the medicalisation of human misery and pain.[15] Taking a similarly hard line is the ancient Greek historian Jason Crowley, who argues that the influence of one's culture can neutralise a combatant's susceptibility to PTSD.[16] Crowley's original argument, which appeared in *Combat Trauma and the Ancient Greeks*, engaged directly with the theory that ancient PTSD existed in the ancient world, but he never considered that combat induced trauma may have manifested differently within those different cultures.

Not all relativist models have been so extreme in their dismissal of PTSD. The work of Edgar Jones et al. has shown that the prevalence

[12] Shay, *Achilles in Vietnam*; J. Shay, *Odysseus in America: Combat Trauma and the Undoing of Character* (New York: Scribner, 2002).

[13] Aislinn Melchior, 'Caesar in Vietnam: Did Roman Soldiers Suffer from Post-traumatic Stress Disorder', *Greece & Rome* 58–2, 2011, 209–23; Jason Crowley, 'Beyond the Universal Soldier: Combat Trauma in Classical Antiquity', in P. Meineck and D. Konstan (eds), *Combat Trauma and the Ancient Greeks* (New York: Palgrave Macmillan, 2014), pp. 105–30; Owen Rees, 'We Need to Talk About Epizelus: PTSD and the Ancient World', *Medical Humanities* 46.1, 2020, 46–54.

[14] Pavlos Ntafoulis, 'A War Psychiatry Approach to Warfare in the Middle Byzantine Period', *History of Psychiatry* 27, 2014, 458–71, accessed at https://doi.org/10.1177/0957154X16663148.

[15] D. Summerfield, 'The Invention of Post-traumatic Stress Disorder and the Social Usefulness of a Psychiatric Category', *British Medical Journal* 322, 2001, 95–8.

[16] Crowley, 'Beyond the Universal Soldier'.

of PTSD in different periods of modern history differs quite dramatically.[17] This raises questions about the expression of trauma within different cultural contexts without dismissing its presence in the historical record. More recently, scholars of the relativist model have considered alternative approaches to historical combat trauma that move away from the medical and scientific reliance that is inherent in the universalist model.[18] But the universalist model is still prevalent, as seen in Łukasz Różycki's recent work on *Battlefield Emotions in Late Antiquity*, in which he claims that the 'Romans understood the phenomenon of post-traumatic stress disorder (PTSD) by war'.[19] Although, notably, the relativist counterargument is not dealt with in any detail.

Medieval and early modern treatment of combat trauma is even more limited, though it is slowly increasing. Medieval studies tend to focus on either physical trauma, such as the injuries sustained on the battlefield,[20] trauma caused by military losses,[21] or war trauma as portrayed in literary

[17] E. Jones, R. Hodgins Vermaas, H. McCartney, C. Beech, I. Palmer, K. Hyams, and S. Wessely, 'Flashbacks and Post-traumatic Stress Disorder: The Genesis of a Twentieth-Century Diagnosis', *British Journal of Psychiatry* 182, 2003, 158–63; E. Jones and S. Wessely, 'War Syndromes: The Impact of Culture on Medically Unexplained Symptoms', *Medical History* 49, 2005, 55–78.

[18] Donna Trembinski, 'Comparing Premodern Melancholy/Mania and Modern Trauma: An Argument in Favour of Historical Experience of Trauma', *History of Psychology* 14, 2011, 80–99; Maurizio Paciaroni and Valentina Arnao, 'Neurology and War: From Antiquity to Modern Times', *Frontiers of Neurology and Neuroscience* 38, 2016, 1–9; Nancy Sherman, 'Moral Injury, Damage, and Repair', in Victor Caston and Silke-Maria Weineck (eds), *Our Ancient Wars: Rethinking War Through the Classics* (Ann Arbor: University of Michigan Press, 2016), pp. 121–54; B. Steinbock, 'Sufferings Too Great for Tears: The Destruction of the Athenian Expeditionary Corps in Sicily', in Melanie Jonasch (ed), *The Fight for Greek Sicily Society, Politics, and Landscape* (Oxford: Oxbow Books, 2020), pp. 73–98.

[19] Łukasz Różycki and Krzysztof Chorzewski (trans), *Battlefield Emotions in Late Antiquity: A Study of Fear and Motivation in Roman Military Treatises* (Leiden: Brill, 2021), pp. 3, 24.

[20] O.H. Creighton, L. Evis, and M. Kingdom, 'The Face of Battle? Debating Arrow Trauma on Medieval Human Remains from Princesshay, Exeter', *The Antiquaries Journal* 100, 2020, 165–89; E. A. Sundman and A. Kjellström, 'Medieval Masculinities and Violence: Weapon-Related Trauma in Skeletal Assemblages from Two Religious Houses in Iceland and Sweden', *European Journal of Archaeology* 23, 2020, 567–84; Wendy J. Turner and Christina Lee (eds), *Trauma in Medieval Society* (Leiden: Brill, 2018).

[21] Megan Cassidy-Welch, 'Grief and Memory After the Battle of Agincourt', in Andrew Villalon and Donald Kagay (eds), *The Hundred Year War (Part II): Different Vistas* (Leiden: Brill, 2008), pp. 133–52.

works.[22] Even when psychological trauma is considered, it is not always done so with reference to the theoretical issues of combat trauma and retrospective diagnosis, with some works taking a general approach to pointing out instances of trauma without reference to trauma theory, and others applying the theory without appreciating the historical context.[23] For pre-modern British history, scholarly treatment of combat trauma tends to fall into the literary, such as in investigations of possible combat trauma as portrayed in Shakespeare—and how this may have been understood by his audiences—or evidence from the British Civil Wars of the seventeenth century.[24]

[22] Raluca Radanescu, 'Emotions and War in Chaucer's Knight's Tale', in Claire McIlroy, Anne M. Scott, and Raluca L. Radulescu (eds), *Literature, Emotions, and Pre-Modern War: Conflict in Medieval and Early Modern Emotion* (Amsterdam: ARC, Amsterdam University Press, 2021), pp. 45–62; Stephanie Downes, Andrew Lynch, and Katrina O'Loughlin (eds), *Emotions and War: Medieval to Romantic Literature* (London: Palgrave, 2015); Stephanie Downes, Andrew Lynch, and Katrina O'Loughlin (eds), *Writing War in Britain and France, 1370–1854: A History of Emotions* (Abingdon: Routledge, 2019); Claire McIlroy and Anne M. Scott (eds), *Literature, Emotions, and Pre-Modern War* (Amsterdam: ARC Humanities Press, 2021).

[23] Katie K. Walker, 'Peril, Flight and the Sad Man: Medieval Theories of the Body in Battle', in Laura Ashe and Ian Patterson (eds), *War and Literature: Essays and Studies* (Cambridge: D. S. Brewer, 2014), pp. 21–37; Craig Taylor, 'Military Courage and Fear in the Late Medieval French Chivalric Imagination', *Cahiers de Recherches Médiévales et Humanistas* 24, 2012, 129–47; Donna Trembinski, 'Comparing Premodern Melancholy/Mania and Modern Trauma: An Argument in Favour of Historical Experience of Trauma', *History of Psychology* 14, 2011, 80–99; Alastair J. MacDonald, 'Courage, Fear and the Experience of the Later Medieval Scottish Soldier', *Scottish Historical Review* XCII, 2013, 176–206; Craig Taylor, *Chivalry and the Ideals of Knighthood in France During the Hundred Years War* (Cambridge: Cambridge University Press, 2013); Thomas Kristian Heebøll-Holm, 'Apocalypse Then? The First Crusade, Traumas of War and Thomas de Marle', in Kerstin Hundahl, Lars Kjaer and Niels Lund (eds), *Denmark and Europe in the Middle Ages c. 1000–1525: Essays in Honour of Professor Michael H. Gelting* (Aldershot: Ashgate, 2014), pp. 237–54; Stephen Spencer, *Emotions in a Crusading Context, 1095–1291* (Oxford: Oxford University Press, 2019); Alan Cooper, '1190, William Longbeard and the Crisis of Angevin England', in Sarah Jones and Sethina Watson (eds), *Christians and Jews in Angevin England: The York Massacre of 1190, Narratives and Contexts* (Woodbridge: Boydell, 2013), pp. 91–105.

[24] Linhan Gan, 'Shakespeare's Clarence: The Medieval Shell-Shocked Soldier', *Critical Survey* 33, 2021, 62–78; Ismini Pells, 'Soliciting Sympathy: The Search for Psychological Trauma in Petitions from Seventeenth-Century Maimed Soldiers', in Erin Peters and Cynthia Richards (eds), *Early Modern Trauma: Europe and the Atlantic World* (Lincoln: University of Nebraska Press, 2021), pp. 129–50; Erin Peters, 'Trauma Narratives of the English Civil War', *Journal for Early Modern Cultural Studies* 16, 2016, 78–94. See also Cynthia Richards, 'Wit and War: The Poetry of John Wilmot and the Trauma of War',

It is important to note that this is a topic that has entered public debate, either as historical research finds its way into the popular press, or journalists and commentators respond to the discussion about combat trauma when it appears in film and television.[25] It has also been widely considered by members of the veteran community, and those who care for them. Works like the Theatre of War Project, and source collections such as that by Meagher and Pryer, show the ways in which historical interpretations of combat trauma are understood outside the historical field.[26] Indeed, considering the historic prevalence of medical researchers to draw upon the pre-modern world to support new theories of combat trauma, and indeed new proposed treatments, then it is not an exaggeration for us to emphasise just how important this debate truly is.[27]

Utilising a number of focused case studies from ancient and medieval Europe, this volume takes an interdisciplinary approach to provide the first edited volume dedicated to the methodological debate that surrounds the usage of post-traumatic stress disorder and combat stress as models to examine the pre-modern world. By publishing chapters that use these

Eighteenth Century Fiction 27, 2014, 25–54; Erin Peters, 'The Deep Staines These Wars Will Leave Behind: Psychological Wounds and Curative Methods in the English Civil Wars', in David Appleby and Andrew Hopper (eds), *Battle-Scarred: Mortality, Medical Care and Military Welfare in the British Civil Wars* (Manchester: Manchester University Press, 2018), pp. 156–73.

[25] Ben Tufft, 'Warriors in Ancient Iraq Suffered Post-traumatic Stress Disorder More than 3,000 Years Ago, Say Researchers', 25 January 2015, *The Independent*, https://www.independent.co.uk/news/science/warriors-ancient-iraq-suffered-post-traumatic-stress-disorder-more-3-000-years-ago-say-researchers-10000953.html, accessed 20 December 21; Erik Brown, 'The Hidden Evidence of PTSD in the Ancient World: The Pain Within the Stories', 3 July 2020, *Medium.com*, https://medium.com/lessons-from-history/the-hidden-evidence-of-ptsd-in-the-ancient-world-eb83752b7d4e, accessed 20 December 21; Anthony Riches, 'Did Roman Soldiers Suffer PTSD?', 29 September 2017, *Historia: Historian of the Historical Writers Association*, http://www.historiamag.com/roman-ptsd/, accessed 20 December 21.

[26] Dan Doyle, 'Most People Don't Realise This Ancient Tale Echoes the Seriousness of PTSD', *The Veterans' Site*, https://blog.theveteranssite.greatergood.com/achilles-ptsd/, accessed 20 December 21; Bryan Doerries, *The Theatre of War: What Ancient Greek Tragedies can Teach Us Today* (London: Scribe, 2016); Brad E. Kelle, *Moral Injury: A Guidebook for Understanding and Engagement* (London: Rowman & Littlefield, 2020), especially Part II; Robert Emmet Meagher and Douglas A. Pryer (eds), *War and Moral Injury: A Reader* (Eugene, OR: Wibf & Stock, 2018); David W. Peters, *Post-traumatic God: How the Church Cares for People Who Have Been to Hell and Back* (New York: Morehouse Publishing, 2016).

[27] Rees, 'We Need To Talk'.

models next to ones that challenge their use, this book offers an open academic discourse on a very popular area of study and, in turn, platforms innovative new directions of research.

The Chapters

The volume opens with three chapters considering combat trauma in the ancient Greek world. Owen Rees begins by discussing some of the issues surrounding the application of psychiatric diagnoses to the historical past, a challenge that is at the core of this collection. He asks how historians can judge psychiatric problems through historical evidence of behaviour when we do not necessarily know what constituted normal behaviour at that time, and thus if events of the past even hold the same diagnostic capabilities. Georgia Proietti follows this by considering 'collective war trauma' in the representations of the Persian wars-related events on the Athenian stage in the immediate aftermath of the war, particularly because of the modern utilisation of classical theatre to aid veterans in coming to terms with combat trauma. Taking Aeschylus' *Persians* (472 BC) as a case study, Proietti argues that theatre and trauma had a different relationship in this period, as performance was used to help the whole community, and not specifically combatants, to come to terms with war. Finally, Constantine Christoforou introduces a script-based approach in his analysis of Sophocles' *Ajax*. This approach emphasises the cultural conditions that influences the hero's behaviour, and in turn Christoforou offers a 'script' for combat trauma within the play.

The study then moves on to Ancient Rome, where Andy Fear looks at legal evidence for PTSD in the Roman army. He argues that these 'dry' texts are in many ways better evidence for trauma than literary sources because of their 'dry' nature: their content was not influenced by rhetorical conventions of the day to the extent that, for example, poetry might have been. They are not, however, without their own issues, and Fear digs into the detail of these texts to demonstrate how they might fruitfully be used. Law is also the focus of Jo Ball's chapter on military suicide. She shows how Hadrian (r. 117–138) created an exception to a law relating to military suicide, in which the dead soldier's goods would be seized, for soldiers who were suffering from physical or mental pain that was considered permanent. The significance of the exemption lies in the way it explicitly recognised the mental and physical toll of warfare.

The final three contributions consider the evidence for combat trauma in the medieval and early modern world. Kathryn Hurlock begins by suggesting Moral Injury as a more flexible and applicable model for understanding war trauma in the past, taking examples from the First Crusade (1096–99) as her case study. She argues that PTSD, being a medical diagnosis, is too rigid for interpreting historical combat trauma, and that historians of all eras would be better served by engaging with the theory of Moral Injury. As moral expectations are culturally, and sometimes individually, specific, the theory can be more clearly and readily applied to a variety of military settings, styles of warfare, and military-related events. Chelsea Grosskopff follows this by exploring evidence for combat trauma in the *Eyrbyggja saga*, a thirteenth-century work about the feud of Snorri Goði and Arnkel Goði. Through this text, she explores Hurlock's suggestion that Moral Injury is a useful theory for analysis, but also considers the figure of the berserker in the text in light of modern studies in trauma physiology and therapy. The volume closes with Ismini Pells' consideration of women and children and the trauma of seventeenth-century Civil War in Britain. Women and children both served in the wars—in a combat capacity and as supporters—and were witnesses and victims of conflict. Here, Pells examines the emotional responses of both women and children as seen in the written record—letters, newsbooks, petitions, diaries, memoirs—to demonstrate what the Civil Wars tell us about their resilience to the trauma of participating in and witnessing combat.

The decision to not include a conclusion was a purposeful one. The aim of this volume is to highlight a variety of historical approaches to the topic of combat stress, many of which contradict or disagree with many others. It is not for this editorial team to draw these approaches together to offer some unifying conclusion. The hope is that this volume will inspire further research, exploring a multitude of possibilities related to our driving question. Maybe then, conclusions can be drawn.

Bibliography

Abdul-Hamid, Walid Khalid, and Jamie Hacker Hughes, 'Nothing New under the Sun: Post-traumatic Stress Disorders in the Ancient World', *Early Science and Medicine* 19.6, 2014, 549–57, accessed at https://doi.org/10.1163/15733823-00196p02.

Brown, Erik, 'The Hidden Evidence of PTSD in the Ancient World: The Pain Within the Stories', 3 July 2020, *Medium.com*, https://medium.com/lessons-from-history/the-hidden-evidence-of-ptsd-in-the-ancient-world-eb83752b7d4e, accessed 20 December 21.

Cassidy-Welch, Megan, 'Grief and Memory After the Battle of Agincourt', in Andrew Villalon and Donald Kagay (eds), *The Hundred Year War (Part II): Different Vistas* (Leiden: Brill, 2008), pp. 133–52.

Caston, Victor, and Silke-Maria Weineck (eds), *Our Ancient Wars: Rethinking War Through the Classics* (Ann Arbor: University of Michigan Press, 2016).

Cooper, Alan, '1190, William Longbeard and the Crisis of Angevin England', in Sarah Jones and Sethina Watson (eds), *Christians and Jews in Angevin England: The York Massacre of 1190, Narratives and Contexts* (Woodbridge: Boydell, 2013), pp. 91–105.

Creighton, O.H., L. Evis, and M. Kingdom, 'The Face of Battle? Debating Arrow Trauma on Medieval Human Remains from Princesshay, Exeter', *The Antiquaries Journal* 100, 2020, 165–89.

Crowley, Jason, 'Beyond the Universal Soldier: Combat Trauma in Classical Antiquity', in P. Meineck and D. Konstan (eds), *Combat Trauma and the Ancient Greeks* (New York: Palgrave Macmillan, 2014), pp. 105–30.

Daly, R.J., 'Samuel Pepys and Post-traumatic Stress Disorder', *British Journal of Psychiatry* 143, 1983, 64–8, accessed at https://doi.org/10.1192/bjp.143.1.64.

Doerries, Bryan, *The Theatre of War: What Ancient Greek Tragedies Can Teach Us Today* (London: Scribe, 2016).

Downes, Stephanie, Andrew Lynch, Katrina O'Loughlin (eds), *Emotions and War: Medieval to Romantic Literature* (London: Palgrave, 2015).

Downes, Stephanie, Andrew Lynch, and Katrina O'Loughlin (eds), *Writing War in Britain and France, 1370-1854: A History of Emotions* (Abingdon: Routledge, 2019).

Doyle, Dan. 'Most People Don't Realise This Ancient Tale Echoes the Seriousness of PTSD', *The Veterans' Site,* https://blog.theveteranssite.greatergood.com/achilles-ptsd/, accessed 20 December 21.

Gan, Linhan, 'Shakespeare's Clarence: The Medieval Shell-Shocked Soldier', *Critical Survey* 33, 2021, 62–78.

Heebøll-Holm, Thomas Kristian, 'Apocalypse Then? The First Crusade, Traumas of War and Thomas de Marle', in Kerstin Hundahl, Lars Kjaer, and Niels Lund (eds), *Denmark and Europe in the Middle Ages c. 1000–1525: Essays in Honour of Professor Michael H. Gelting* (Aldershot: Ashgate, 2014), pp. 237–54.

James, Sharon L., 'The Battered Shield: Survivor's Guilt and Family Trauma in Menander's Aspis', in Peter Meineck and David Konstan (eds), *Combat Trauma and the Ancient Greeks* (New York: Palgrave Macmillan, 2014), pp. 237–60.

Jones, Edgar, and Simon Wessely, 'War Syndromes: The Impact of Culture on Medically Unexplained Symptoms', *Medical History* 49, 2005, 55–78.

Jones, Edgar, Robert Hodgins Vermaas, Helen McCartney, Charlotte Beech, Ian Palmer, Kenneth Hyams, and Simon Wessely, 'Flashbacks and Post-traumatic Stress Disorder: The Genesis of a Twentieth-Century Diagnosis', *British Journal of Psychiatry* 182, 2003, 158–63.

Kelle, Brad E., *Moral Injury: A Guidebook for Understanding and Engagement* (London: Rowman & Littlefield, 2020).

MacDonald, Alastair J., 'Courage, Fear and the Experience of the Later Medieval Scottish Soldier', *Scottish Historical Review* XCII, 2013, 176–206.

Macowiak, Philip A., 'Post-traumatic Stress Reactions before the Advent of Post-traumatic Stress Disorder: Potential Effects on the Lives and Legacies of Alexander the Great, Captain James Cook, Emily Dickinson, and Florence Nightingale', *Military Medicine* 173, 2008, 1158–63, accessed at https://doi.org/10.7205/milmed.173.12.1158.

McIlroy, Claire and Anne M. Scott (eds), *Literature, Emotions, and Pre-Modern War* (Amsterdam: ARC Humanities Press, 2021).

Meagher, Robert Emmet, and Douglas A. Pryer (eds), *War and Moral Injury: A Reader* (Eugene, OR: Wibf & Stock, 2018).

Meineck, Peter, 'Combat Trauma and the Tragic Stage: Ancient Culture and Modern Catharsis?', in Victor Caston and Silke-Maria Weineck (eds), *Our Ancient Wars: Rethinking War Through the Classics* (Ann Arbor: University of Michigan Press, 2016), pp. 184–208.

Meineck, Peter, and David Konstan (eds), *Combat Trauma and the Ancient Greeks* (New York: Palgrave Macmillan, 2014).

Melchior, Aislinn, 'Caesar in Vietnam: Did Roman Soldiers Suffer from Post-traumatic Stress Disorder', *Greece & Rome* 58-2, 2011, 209–23.

Monoson, S.S., 'Socrates in Combat: Trauma and Resilience in Plato's Political Theory', in P. Meineck and D. Konstan (eds), *Combat Trauma and the Ancient Greeks* (New York: Palgrave Macmillan, 2014), pp. 131–62.

Morris, Alexandra F., 'Alexander the Great: Head to Head with CTW (Chronic Traumatic Encephalopathy)', *Athens Journal of History* 3, 1983, 225–34, accessed at https://doi.org/10.30958/ajhis.3-3-3.

Ntafoulis, Pavlos, 'A War Psychiatry Approach to Warfare in the Middle Byzantine Period', *History of Psychiatry* 27, 2014, 458–71, accessed at https://doi.org/10.1177/0957154X16663148.

Paciaroni, Maurizio, and Valentina Arnao, 'Neurology and War: From Antiquity to Modern Times', *Frontiers of Neurology and Neuroscience* 38, 2016, 1–9.

Pells, Ismini, 'Soliciting Sympathy: The Search for Psychological Trauma in Petitions from Seventeenth-Century Maimed Soldiers', in Erin Peters and Cynthia Richards (eds), *Early Modern Trauma: Europe and the Atlantic World* (Lincoln: University of Nebraska Press, 2021), pp. 129–50.

Peters, David W., *Post-traumatic God: How the Church Cares for People Who Have Been to Hell and Back* (New York: Morehouse Publishing, 2016).

Peters, Erin, 'Trauma Narratives of the English Civil War', *Journal for Early Modern Cultural Studies* 16, 2016, 78–94.

Peters, Erin, 'The Deep Staines These Wars Will Leave Behind': Psychological Wounds and Curative Methods in the English Civil Wars', in David Appleby and Andrew Hopper (eds), *Battle-Scarred: Mortality, Medical Care and Military Welfare in the British Civil Wars* (Manchester: Manchester University Press, 2018), pp. 156–73.

Proietti, Giorgia, 'Athens as a "Landscape of Trauma": Phrynichus' Sack of Miletus and the Aftermath of the Persian Wars', in Lucia Cecchet, Christopher Degelmann, and Maik Patzelt (eds), *The Ancient War's Impact on the Home Front* (Newcastle-upon-Tyne: Cambridge Scholars, 2019), pp. 79–98.

Raaflaub, Kurt, 'Lysistrata and War's Impact on the Home Front', in Victor Caston and Silke-Maria Weineck (eds), *Our Ancient Wars: Rethinking War Through the Classics* (Ann Arbor: University of Michigan Press, 2016), pp. 38–74.

Radanescu, Raluca, 'Emotions and War in Chaucer's Knight's Tale', in Claire McIlroy, Anne M. Scott, and Raluca L. Radulescu (eds), *Literature, Emotions, and Pre-Modern War: Conflict in Medieval and Early Modern Emotion* (Amsterdam: ARC, Amsterdam University Press, 2021), pp. 45–62.

Rees, O., 'We Need to Talk About Epizelus: PTSD and the Ancient World', *Medical Humanities* 46.1, 2020, 46–54.

Richards, Cynthia, 'Wit and War: The Poetry of John Wilmot and the Trauma of War', *Eighteenth Century Fiction* 27, 2014, 25–54.

Riches, Anthony, 'Did Roman Soldiers Suffer PTSD?', 29 September 2017, *Historia: Historian of the Historical Writers Association*, http://www.historiamag.com/roman-ptsd/, accessed 20 December 21.

Różycki, Łukasz and Krzysztof Chorzewski (trans), *Battlefield Emotions in Late Antiquity: A Study of Fear and Motivation in Roman Military Treatises* (Leiden: Brill, 2021).

Shay, J., *Achilles in Vietnam: Trauma and the Undoing of Character* (New York: Athenaeum, 1994).

Shay, J., *Odysseus in America: Combat Trauma and the Undoing of Character* (New York: Scribner, 2002).

Sherman, Nancy, '"He Gave Me His Hand But Took My Bow": Trust and Trustworthiness in the Philoctetes and Our Wars', in Peter Meineck and David Konstan (eds), *Combat Trauma and the Ancient Greeks* (New York: Palgrave Macmillan, 2014), pp. 207–24.

Sherman, Nancy, 'Moral Injury, Damage, and Repair', in Victor Caston and Silke-Maria Weineck (eds), *Our Ancient Wars: Rethinking War Through the Classics* (Ann Arbor: University of Michigan Press, 2016), pp. 121–54.

Sorkin Rabinowitz, Nancy, 'Women and War in Tragedy', in Peter Meineck and David Konstan (eds), *Combat Trauma and the Ancient Greeks* (New York: Palgrave Macmillan, 2014), pp. 207–25.

Spencer, Stephen, *Emotions in a Crusading Context, 1095-1291* (Oxford: Oxford University Press, 2019).

Steinbock, B., 'Sufferings Too Great for Tears': The Destruction of the Athenian Expeditionary Corps in Sicily', in Melanie Jonasch (ed), *The Fight for Greek Sicily Society, Politics, and Landscape* (Oxford: Oxbow Books, 2020), pp. 73–98.

Summerfield, Derek, 'The Invention of Post-traumatic Stress Disorder and the Social Usefulness of a Psychiatric Category', *British Medical Journal* 322, 2001, 95–8.

Sundman, E.A., and A. Kjellström, 'Medieval Masculinities and Violence: Weapon-Related Trauma in Skeletal Assemblages from Two Religious Houses in Iceland and Sweden', *European Journal of Archaeology* 23, 2020, 567–84.

Taylor, Craig, 'Military Courage and Fear in the Late Medieval French Chivalric Imagination', *Cahiers de Recherches Médiévales et Humanistas* 24, 2012, 129–47.

Taylor, Craig, *Chivalry and the Ideals of Knighthood in France During the Hundred Years War* (Cambridge: Cambridge University Press, 2013).

Trembinski, Donna, 'Comparing Premodern Melancholy/Mania and Modern Trauma: An Argument in Favour of Historical Experience of Trauma', *History of Psychology* 14, 2011, 80–99.

Tritle, L., *Melos to My Lai* (London: Routledge, 2000).

Tritle, Lawrence, 'Gorgias, the Encomium of Helen, and the Trauma of War', *Clio's Psyche* 16.2, 2009, 195–9.

Tritle, Lawrence, '"Ravished Minds" in the Ancient World', in Peter Meineck and David Konstan (eds), *Combat Trauma and the Ancient Greeks* (New York: Palgrave Macmillan, 2014), pp. 87–104.

Tufft, Ben, 'Warriors in Ancient Iraq Suffered Post-traumatic Stress Disorder more than 3,000 years ago, say researchers', 25 January 2015, *The Independent,* https://www.independent.co.uk/news/science/warriors-ancient-iraq-suffered-post-traumatic-stress-disorder-more-3-000-years-ago-say-researchers-10000953.html accessed 20 December 2021.

Turner, Wendy J., and Christina Lee (eds), *Trauma in Medieval Society* (Leiden: Brill, 2018).

Walker, Katie K., 'Peril, Flight and the Sad Man: Medieval Theories of the Body in Battle', in Laura Ashe and Ian Patterson (eds), *War and Literature: Essays and Studies* (Cambridge: D. S. Brewer, 2014), pp. 21–37.

Post-traumatic Stress Disorder: An Ancient Greek Case Study in Retrospective Diagnosis

Owen Rees

The desire to impose modern experience upon the past, and modern medical understanding through the form of retrospective diagnosis, is a long-standing trend. Most commonly, we see this in the study of biological disease, with many medical scholars looking to label a disease or plague in the past.[1] What is perhaps slightly less common, but still in possession of a centuries-long tradition, is the inclination to read the

[1] For discussion on this field of scholarship, and its tradition, see A. Cunningham, 'Identifying Disease in the Past: Cutting the Gordian Knot', *Asclepio* 54, 2002, 13–34; J. Arrizabalaga, 'Problematizing Retrospective Diagnosis in the History of Disease', *Asclepio* 54, 2002, 51–70; K.H. Leven, '"At Times These Ancient Facts Seem to Lie Before Me Like a Patient on a Hospital Bed"—Retrospective Diagnosis and Ancient Medical History', in Manfred Horstmanshoff and Marten Stol (eds), *Magic and Rationality in Ancient Near Eastern and Graeco-Roman Medicine* (Leiden: Brill, 2004), pp. 369–86; A. Karenberg and F.P. Moog, 'Next Emperor Please! No End to Retrospective Diagnosis', *Journal of the History of the Neurosciences* 13.2, 2004, 143–49.

O. Rees (✉)
Department of History, Politics and Philosophy, Manchester Metropolitan University, Manchester, UK
e-mail: O.rees@mmu.ac.uk

O. Rees et al. (eds.), *Combat Stress in Pre-modern Europe*, Mental Health in Historical Perspective,
https://doi.org/10.1007/978-3-031-09947-2_2

historic source material and diagnose individuals with mental illnesses.[2] Of these, the diagnosis of schizophrenia has aroused the most attention, with many scholars claiming its existence in the pre-modern world while sceptics have challenged this claim in no uncertain terms.[3] However, the scholarly discussion surrounding the very nature of this psychological retrospective diagnosis, and how it differs in nature to that of biological disease, is still underdeveloped.

The reliance on modern medicine to understand the pre-modern world presupposes that medicine is in some way a 'hard science' that possesses an element of universal truth which can be transplanted into any time period and any culture. Yet, medicine is not a 'hard science'; it is a product of the socio-cultural environment in which it was created. Additionally, this approach assumes that the historic evidence is offering symptomology in its descriptions of events or behaviours, yet many of these writers had no medical training, and we do not know if they recorded things that were relevant to the central issue or were simply considered of importance to the lay-author. In essence, as we read the texts, it is impossible to deduce whether we are receiving relevant data for a diagnosis or not.

These problems become exponentially more complicated when we consider mental illnesses or diagnoses, rather than those seen as biological. The issue was articulated by Erwin Ackerknecht in 1943, in his critique on the contemporary trend of diagnosing Amazonian tribesmen with schizophrenia, when he observed that:

> A man, e.g., with paranoid behaviour and ideas, unlike a man suffering with tuberculosis, may in another cultural set-up where almost everybody

[2] C. Thumiger, *A History of the Mind and Mental Health in Classical Greek Medical Thought* (Cambridge: Cambridge University Press, 2017), pp. 2–8.

[3] N.M. Bark, 'On the History of Schizophrenia: Evidence of Its Existence Before 1800', *New York State Journal of Medicine* 88.7, 1988, 374–83; C.V. Haldipur, 'Madness in Ancient India: Concept of Insanity in Charaka Samhita (first century A.D.)', *Comprehensive Psychiatry* 25.3, 1984, 335–44; D.V. Jeste, R. del Carmen, J.B. Lohr, and R.J. Wyatt, 'Did Schizophrenia Exist Before the Eighteenth Century?', *Comprehensive Psychiatry* 26.6, 1985, 493–503; K. Otsuka and A. Sakai, 'Haizmann's Madness: The Concept of Bizarreness and the Diagnosis of Schizophrenia', *History of Psychiatry* 15.1, 2004, 73–82; M.H. Stone, *Healing the Mind: A History of Psychiatry from Antiquity to the Present* (New York: W. W. Norton, 1997); H.A. Youssef and F.A. Youssef, 'Evidence for the Existence of Schizophrenia in Medieval Islamic Society', *History of Psychiatry* 7, 1996, 55–62; D. Fraguas, 'Problems with Retrospective Studies of the Presence of Schizophrenia', *History of Psychiatry* 20.1, 2009, 61–71.

> shares his attitude, be by no means socially disabled, but a normal and ideal participant of his society.[4]

The presentation of atypicality is not, in and of itself, enough to validate a universal diagnosis. Disability theorists have rightly highlighted the importance of functionality in regard to atypical presentations.[5] If a person is able to function unimpaired within their society, then they do not attract any attempt to explain the differences that are observable. Only when atypicality is at odds with societal norms and values, when it impairs the ability to function adequately within the social framework, does it become observed, qualified, diagnosed, and often stigmatised.

Psychiatric diagnoses frequently emphasise behavioural symptoms; this in turn gives historians a twofold problem: (1) Can we know whether these behavioural symptoms are predominantly characteristic of our own social normality, and thus their observation by clinicians confirms simply antithetical and undesirous behaviours in the modern day? (2) Like Ackerknecht, we must ask: if those same behaviours appeared in another cultural sphere, do they still hold the same diagnostic capabilities? That is to say, do the sources tell us about this behaviour because it is abnormal and thus potentially symptomatic of an issue, or for another reason? This chapter will focus on one such diagnosis, post-traumatic stress disorder, and address some of the pressing methodological issues surrounding such a practice.

Approaches in Retrospective PTSD Studies

The study of PTSD in the ancient world has been well covered in the Introduction, but the tradition stretches back further than Dr Jonathan Shay. As early as 1919, medical scholars have asked whether the ancient sources offer accounts of war neuroses.[6] Over the past century, the name of the diagnosis assigned has changed. It began with discussing ancient

[4] Erwin H. Ackerknecht, 'Psychopathology, Primitive Medicine and Primitive Culture', *Bulletin of the History of Medicine* 14.1, 1943, 37.

[5] E. DePoy and S.F. Gilson, *Studying Disability: Multiple Theories and Responses* (London: Sage, 2011), pp. 9–10, 96–97; Dana Lee Baker, *The Politics of Neurodiversity: Why Public Policy Matters* (Boulder: Lynne Reiner, 2011), pp. 12–5.

[6] O. Rees, 'We Need to Talk About Epizelus: PTSD and the Ancient World', *Medical Humanities* 46.1, 2020, 46.

cases of shell shock, then commentators used other terms such as conversion disorder, hysteria, war neurosis, and the modern term PTSD. This mixture of psychiatric diagnosis and vague psychoanalytical labelling is indicative of the nature of the ailment.

PTSD is defined in psychological terms as a 'disorder of traumatic memory', and associated symptoms such as intrusive memories and flashbacks lead to symptomatic behavioural changes such as avoidance of the traumatic memory.[7] According to the most prominent model of diagnosis set out within the *Diagnostics and Statistical Manual of Mental Disorders-5*, the designation requires that the patient fulfils eight requirements. As a fundamental requirement for the modern diagnosis, it is always within these criteria that historical attempts of retrospective diagnosis fall apart. This *splitting* approach to ancient retrospective diagnosis is an impossibility.[8] It is so difficult to identify all of the criteria in the ancient source material that leading proponents of the universalist model usually end up abandoning the clinical definition.[9] But if we ignore the clinical definitions of PTSD, what exactly are we doing by discussing PTSD in the pre-modern world?

For example, Lawrence Tritle produced a thorough case study of PTSD in his analysis of the fifth-century BC Spartan commander Clearchus. In his groundbreaking analysis, Tritle did not disguise the fact that the clinical definition of PTSD was too limiting for ancient military historians:

> It should be noted that this list of characteristics differs slightly from those listed in the *Diagnostics and Statistical Manual of Mental Disorders* ... I follow Shay here, as his analysis of PTSD includes the ideas of betrayal and destruction of social trust, whereas the DSM list omits these and refers to such traits as the avoidance of thoughts, feelings, etc.

The model Tritle was following was laid out in Shay's seminal work in 1994, so it is at least worth noting that from the very beginning of this historical discussion, the diagnosis of PTSD, and thus a *splitting*

[7] Edgar Jones and Simon Wessely, 'War Syndromes: The Impact of Culture on Medically Unexplained Symptoms', *Medical History* 49, 2005, 56.

[8] D. Fraguas, 'Problems with Retrospective Studies of the Presence of Schizophrenia', *History of Psychiatry* 20.1, 2009, 62.

[9] J. Shay, *Achilles in Vietnam* (New York: Athenaeum, 1994), pp. 166–69; L. Tritle, *Melos to My Lai* (London: Routledge, 2000), pp. 57–8.

approach to the diagnosis, was not a fruitful arena for analysis. This is of little surprise, considering that Dr Shay was already formulating his new model of Moral Injury as a means to better understand the experience of veterans.[10] However, Shay's original supposition has created an environment in which historians have used the clinical label of PTSD as a means to validate the problematic practice of cherry-picking symptoms from the definition laid out in the *DSM*. This *lumping* approach means that scholars search for more general signs of madness, emotional distress, or behavioural patterns that can be related to a combat experience.[11] To take the example of Clearchus, whose behaviour as described in Xenophon's *Anabasis* is best described as severe and at times brutal, Tritle argues that this behavioural shift is best explained by the trauma of his combat experience. The explanation is a fascinating one, and may well be correct, but there is one fundamental issue that such a claim must face—the time frame. In the *DSM*, one of the criteria for PTSD—or in the case of Clearchus complex PTSD—is the symptomatological time frame. Criteria E requires that the behavioural effects need to have begun or indeed worsened after the trauma, and Criteria F requires symptoms to have lasted for more than one month. However, we do not have any account of Clearchus' life before 412 BC, at which time he was already 39 years old. In effect, we do not know if combat, or any other form of trauma, was responsible for this behavioural pattern; he could have always been that way. Being a violent, arrogant, and socially isolated man does not demand the need for a diagnosis; not on its own, anyway.

This *lumping* approach has removed the analytical focus from the defining features of PTSD, and has allowed for the continued confusion between what is symptomatic of trauma and what is not. A prime example would be the observation of stress reactions in historic protagonists. Shay's own work focused on the experience of Achilles and used a psychological and neurological understanding of combat stress reactions to explore the hero's experience in combat. This has since become a model by which to explore ancient trauma, which is not what Shay

[10] J. Shay, 'Moral Injury', *Intertexts* 16.1, 2012, 57–66.

[11] D. Fraguas, 'Problems with Retrospective Studies of the Presence of Schizophrenia', *History of Psychiatry* 20.1, 2009, 63.

intended.[12] Combat stress reactions, often simplified to 'fight, flight or freeze', do not prove the presence of trauma. Shay never claims that the 'berserker' state of Achilles proves he had PTSD, but it does give us a more nuanced understanding of what is poetic hyperbole, and what may reflect a reality of combat.

If we are to continue discussing the PTSD-like symptoms potentially present in the ancient evidence, it is vital that we acknowledge the inherent issues in our source material. We must also accept that, contrary to our popular model which considers psychiatric medicine as almost a 'hard science', the classification of mental disorders is unequivocally rooted in, and shaped by, cultural factors.[13] In effect, we must be honest in what we are actually discussing, because it no longer represents the clinical definition of PTSD.

Presentism in Retrospectively Diagnosing PTSD

Retrospective diagnosis is, by its very nature, steeped in presentism. The majority of our sources are not offering us symptoms to be read as a diagnosis, and those that are, such as the Hippocratic Corpus, are offering symptoms deemed relevant within their own medical framework. Considering that the Greek world of the fifth and fourth centuries BC did not separate physical and psychological processing, symptoms of *mania* are frequently associated with physical manifestations.[14] A similar methodological issue arises from the classical Greek vagueness when it comes to defining mental illnesses, or psychological symptoms of related illnesses. The recent work by Chiara Thumiger, on the Greek vocabulary of insanity, highlights the multifaceted symptoms that are situated under umbrella terms like *mania* and *melancholia*.[15] Therefore, even to read that a historic figure was melancholic does not constitute a firmly

[12] In his follow up book *Odysseus in America*, 149, he makes the observation that combat adaptations may account of the symptoms of PTSD in the *DSM*, but equally advised his readers to go and read the list of symptoms themselves.

[13] G.E. Berrios, 'Classifications in Psychiatry: A Conceptual History', *Australian and New Zealand Journal of Psychiatry* 33.2, 1999, 145–60.

[14] C. Thumiger, *A History of the Mind and Mental Health in Classical Greek Medical Thought* (Cambridge: Cambridge University Press), pp. 72–3.

[15] C. Thumiger, 'The Early Greek Medical Vocabulary of Insanity', in William V. Harris (ed), *Mental Disorders in the Classical World* (Leiden: Brill, 2013), pp. 61–4.

defined symptom. This observation is not a modern phenomenon, and was frequently used as a critique of classical Greek medicine during the Roman Imperial period.[16]

Thus, we must unpick the evidence to decide whether a particular source is offering us a symptom, what that symptom actually is, and whether that is a true observation or indicative of the socio-medical environment which is making the observation. To put it bluntly, unless the evidence comes through a medical observer, and those observations come with clear patterns of behaviour and symptomology, the experience of the individual cannot be considered pathological; yet this is precisely how we are judging it.

So what does this mean for our evidence? Are we seeing the wood from the trees by noting these manifested symptoms of an understood diagnosis? Or are we in effect changing the evidence, modifying it to suit our own end? As Fraguas astutely noted, using Heisenberg's uncertainty principle: 'it is conceivable that the study of antiquity involves such a change; the original source is modified by the observational process itself'.[17] By forcing our understanding of the mind, of trauma, and of the experience of the modern veteran onto our source material, we are looking at it through a filter and therefore not seeing what the source material is actually telling us about those same experiences. There is no question that there is evidence for a behavioural and psychological impact on the ancient individual following his or her experience of war. But that does not mean that it would, nor indeed should, look the same as it does in the modern day.

Trauma must be a negative experience, and as a result context matters. Considering the modern military experience, a psychological state of vigilance, of explosive aggression, and of emotional numbing in the face of a combat threat can be the difference between life and death. As such, evidence for combat stress reactions can never stand alone as evidence of trauma. They are evolutionary adaptions that the human being must undergo to survive. However, if those behaviours continue into civilian life, we have what Shay describes as one of the 'key symptoms of PTSD

[16] Aretaeus of Cappadocia, *On Chronic Diseases*, 1.6; Aetius, *Iatrika*, 6.8; W.V. Harris, 'Thinking About Mental Disorders in Classical Antiquity', in William V. Harris (ed), *Mental Disorders in the Classical World* (Leiden: Brill, 2013), pp. 1–2.

[17] D. Fraguas, 'Problems with Retrospective Studies of the Presence of Schizophrenia', *History of Psychiatry* 20.1, 2009, 64.

and of the personality changes that mark its severe forms'.[18] The context of those behaviours, and how they are received by the wider society, equally determines the impact on the individual. This is why the presentist imposition of retrospective diagnosis is restrictive to our understanding of the ancient world. Innate within this form of study is the precept that the diagnosis is the universal phenomenon, not the experience: in other words, that it is not the psychological impact of war on the individual that manifests in all time periods and in all cultures, but specifically PTSD.[19]

Even if we identify PTSD-like symptoms in the historical record, this does not equate to finding PTSD. A diagnosis and the experience of the diagnosis are not the same thing. One may share the symptoms in different time periods, but conceptions of military service, of 'madness' and illness more generally, and of the socio-religious understanding of the human experience, strongly influence the manifestation of those symptoms. If these PTSD-like symptoms offer a different experience for our historical subjects, then it is very hard to argue that they are evidence for PTSD.[20]

Modern Disorder or Historical Constant?

Few elements of this retrospective diagnosis are more controversial than the question of its modernity. Pioneered by the anthropologist Allan Young, proponents of PTSD being a modern disorder claim that PTSD is not timeless, and the idea of traumatic memory is an experiential concept that exists no earlier than the nineteenth century.[21] Such a view has been criticised, not least by Tritle, as being ignorant of the ancient

[18] J. Shay, *Achilles in Vietnam: Trauma and the Undoing of Character* (New York: Athenaeum, 1994), xx.

[19] This pan-cultural, universalist model has led at least one team of researchers to use the ancient world to argue that the same is true of treatment: 'it indicates that modern Western approaches to the psychological treatment of trauma are not entirely culturally dependent and may be applied to the treatment of trauma with patients from different cultural traditions.'—Y. Ustinova and E. Cardeña, 'Combat Stress Disorders and Their Treatment in Ancient Greece', *Psychological Trauma: Theory, Research, Practice, and Policy* 6.6, 2014, 746.

[20] For a historical case study that examines the differing reception of the 'traumatised' warrior, see O. Rees, 'We Need to Talk About Epizelus: PTSD and the Ancient World', *Medical Humanities* 46.1, 2020, 46–54.

[21] A. Young, *The Harmony of Illusions* (Princeton: Princeton University Press, 1995).

evidence which seems to clearly show traumatic memory, and traumatic re-experiencing, by figures such as Odysseus.

Young is not alone in his assertion. Psychiatrist Kirmayer proposed that different, non-Western cultures witness a different symptomatic outcome based on trauma; that even in the modern day, trauma is not a universally observable phenomenon with a select list of symptoms and characteristics based on cause and effect, which in turn 'ignores the social and cultural embedding of distress that ensures that trauma, loss, and restitution are inextricably intertwined'.[22] Bracken agrees with Kirmayer and argues that PTSD needs to be seen as the product of not simply trauma but '*trauma and culture* acting together'.[23] Edgar Jones' study on one specific symptom of PTSD highlights this further still. He examined randomised records of UK servicemen who had been awarded pensions for post-combat disorders, from 1854 onwards, for evidence of flashbacks. He found that the symptom becomes more apparent in diagnoses after the Second World War, whereas servicemen before this period emphasised more somatic symptoms.

Such an approach raises serious questions of historical continuity for the phenomenon of war-induced trauma. Universalist suggestions of continuity are neatly surmised in O'Brien's critique of the position, that 'PTSD is merely the renaming or the synthesis of an age-old condition'.[24] But the growing realisation that trauma cannot be separated from the culture of the individual experiencing it means that we can no longer use such over simplifications. If symptoms look the same, it is because of our own perception of trauma; to truly understand a historical case of trauma, it is essential to remove ourselves from the modern diagnostic parameters and see how trauma and culture manifest within the source material.

The discussion is problematic, not least because of the disparity in medical contexts between the present and the ancient past. The very

[22] L.J. Kirmayer, 'Confusion of the Senses: Implications of Ethnocultural Variations in Somatoform and Dissociative Disorders for PTSD', in A.J. Marsella, M.J. Friedman, E.T. Gerrity, and R.M. Scurfield (eds), *Ethnocultural Aspects of Posttraumatic Stress Disorder: Issues, Research, and Clinical Applications* (Washington, DC: American Psychological Association, 1996), p. 150.

[23] P.J. Bracken, 'Post-modernity and Post-traumatic Stress Disorder', *Social Science & Medicine* 53.6, 2001, 742.

[24] S. O'Brien, *Traumatic Events and Mental Health* (Cambridge: Cambridge University Press, 1998), p. 5.

notion of trauma presupposes a separation between the mind and the body, so to speak. To ancient writers, there was no clear distinction between somatic and psychological causes for diseases.[25] This lack of distinction is being emulated by the universalist use of neurobiology as the underpinning of their methodology, in effect trying to reassert the somatic element of trauma into the discussion. But this approach emphasises the diagnosis as the source of information, guided as it must be by the modern medical studies that are then adapted to fit the ancient source material.

Other models are being used in historical studies that approach this question from a different perspective, not one of diagnosis but of phenomenology. Key among them is the subject of Moral Injury (see Hurlock in this volume). This has the advantage of removing the analysis from a diagnosis that is entangled within social parameters of accepted behaviours and norms, and medical understanding. However, it still has the potential to exude a common set of moral parameters throughout a wide chronological and societal spectrum. It is imperative that the commonality is identified, and all else is contextualised within its own time period and cultural framework. The core commonality, the central phenomenon under investigation, is predominantly the psychological impact that war and military service can have on an individual, either in service or after their transition back to civilian life—what we might call combat trauma. Ideally, this should be split into two different, albeit at times intersecting issues: the impact of war on the individual, and the issues the individual experiences in transition from military service to civilian life.

Interpreting PTSD-Like Symptoms in Ancient Texts

PTSD is a disorder defined by its aetiology; there needs to be a traumatic experience or stressor to which the person was exposed, whether directly or indirectly. As the historical debate still focuses on combat-induced PTSD, it can be assumed that combat offers such an exposure.

[25] N. Metzger, 'Railway Spine, Shell-shock and Psychological Trauma: The Limits of Retrospective Diagnosis', in Eve-Marie Becker, Jan Dochhorn, Else Holt (eds), *Trauma and Traumatization in Individual and Collective Dimensions: Insights from Biblical Studies and Beyond* (Gottingen: Vandenhoek & Ruprecht GmBH, 2014), p. 56.

This idea has been challenged by Jason Crowley, who argues that the Classical Athenian hoplite was culturally immunised from the effect of war, which may impact the likelihood of experiencing PTSD thereafter.[26] His argument is appealing, but it only compares the hoplite to the modern diagnostic construct of PTSD, and does not consider the possibility of a general phenomenon of warfare having an impact on the behaviour of combatants after war. Indeed, it is noticeable that his seminal work on this topic neglects to deal with any of the direct evidence of PTSD-like symptoms offered by the likes of Tritle. So, while Crowley rightly shows how the experience of the modern and ancient combatants cannot, and should not, be compared, he does not prove that Athenian hoplites were immunised from other possible causes of trauma, nor that that trauma may manifest very differently within each culture. To that end, the negative attribution to war, even in a polemic culture like Athens, suggests that the experience of war was not a nice one, and could leave an indelible mark on the individual.[27]

As a result of this aetiological foundation to PTSD, it is necessary for any symptoms being collated to be shown to relate to a military experience first and foremost, but not all studies have been able to achieve this. There has been a lot of media interest in the article of W.K. Abdul-Hamid and J.H. Hughes, who have argued that the Assyrian medical texts 'document symptoms of post-traumatic stress disorders'.[28] Yet, the examples used fail to identify the experience of war as the cause of their symptoms. In fact, the modern editors of the manual used by Abdul-Hamid and Hughes actually describe the difficulty of separating evidence for different types of shock symptoms and the origins of that shock.[29] Furthermore, Abdul-Hamid and Hughes make no mention of the importance of three days in the Assyrian symptomology. The three instances identified in the

[26] Jason Crowley, 'Beyond the Universal Soldier: Combat Trauma in Classical Antiquity', in P. Meineck and D. Konstan (eds), *Combat Trauma and the Ancient Greeks* (New York: Palgrave Macmillan, 2014), p. 117.

[27] See for instance Thucydides, *History of the Peloponnesian War* 2.8, and similar sentiments expressed in the works of poets such as Pindar, fr. 110.

[28] Walid Khalid Abdul-Hamid and Jamie Hacker Hughes, 'Nothing New under the Sun: Post-traumatic Stress Disorders in the Ancient World', *Early Science and Medicine* 19.6, 2014, 549–57.

[29] J. Scurlock and Burton Anderson, *Diagnoses in Assyrian and Babylonian Medicine* (Chicago: University of Illinois Press, 2005), p. 349.

manual, and covered in the paper, each reference the duration of the symptoms to three days.[30] If we are to accept the described symptoms as an accurate observation, are we not also bound to accept the duration as well? According to the *DSM-5*, PTSD symptoms need to last for at least a month and there is simply no evidence that this was the case. In this instance, they are evidence of a phenomenon, but not the PTSD diagnosis.

But this is a rare case, particularly when looking at claims of PTSD in the ancient Greek world. The prolificacy of combat experience in Greek culture makes the identification of the aetiology of symptoms quite simple, although as Christoforou points out in his chapter, sometimes the aetiology is not given as war, no matter how much we want it to be. Using the ***lumping*** approach, it *is* possible to identify a historical agent with clear military service exhibiting possible symptoms. Having done that, we are now faced with a common historical issue: the conflation of language. While the term PTSD does not exist in the ancient Greek language, it is possible for them to still describe the disorder in their own terms.[31] To avoid the presentist issues discussed above, it is important to not only identify the terminology that may reflect symptoms but also identify how that author, and other authors, use that terminology in other instances. We must not only contextualise the word within its own culture, but also within the syntax of the specific author.

To use a prominent example, we may return to Clearchus the Spartan. One of the important aspects of his biography, given in a eulogistic form by Xenophon, is his description as a *philopolemos* (war-lover). To Tritle, such a personality trait was in need of answering:

> The question that arises is why men like Clearchus and his counterparts in Vietnam and the Western Front became so entranced with violence. The answer is to be found in the natural 'high' that violence induces in those exposed to it, and in the PTSD that follows this exposure.[32]

Yet, to echo the words of Aislinn Melchior, the very fact that we feel the need to answer this question shows the cultural chasm that exists between

[30] Ibid., p. 351.

[31] L. Tritle, *Melos to My Lai* (London: Routledge, 2000), p. 59.

[32] Ibid., p. 56.

ourselves and the classical Greek world.[33] The word does not appear in any of Xenophon's other texts, but it does appear as an epithet in Homer's *Iliad* no less than ten times.[34] The obviously positive connotations of these epithets is undermined somewhat by Diodorus Siculus' usage to describe another Spartan, the king Agesilaus, in contrast to his partner king Agesipolis who is described as peaceful and just.[35] Diodorus' usage suggests an innate personality trait in Agesilaus as opposed to a shift in his behaviour. Such a trait is also reflected in Plutarch's *Life of Agesiluas*, where he describes the king with three adjectives: violent (βίαιος), stubborn (ἀτενής), and greedy of war (ἄπληστος).[36] This usage to describe an innate characteristic is confirmed by another instance, when Diodorus uses the word *philopolemos* to describe the Thebans as a people.[37] Furthermore, we see Diodorus use the antonym to describe Artaxerxes II (οὐκ ὢν φιλοπόλεμος), a trait he specifically associates with military failure.[38] So, while it could be argued that being a *philopolemos* was not always a positive attribute, not being one also led to criticism.

The issue with the term *philopolemos* is that it is not a diagnostic term. Xenophon is not offering a symptom, he is trying to explain the behaviour of Clearchus as he saw fit. As Roisman observes, the character painted in the eulogy does not accurately reflect his actions in the earlier episodes of the *Anabasis*.[39] Furthermore, Clearchus is described as choosing a life of war over one of peace.[40] The characterisation Xenophon gives is not one to explain Clearchus' behaviour as a man, which comes later in the eulogy; this label is used to explain why he never retired from war. While it may be tempting to align this with a modern notion of an addiction to combat, such an addiction necessitates that combat was considered a

[33] Aislinn Melchior, 'Caesar in Vietnam: Did Roman Soldiers Suffer from Post-traumatic Stress Disorder', *Greece & Rome* 58.2, 2011, 216.

[34] Homer, *Iliad* 16.65; 16.90; 16.836; 17.194; 17.224; 19.269; 20.351; 21.86; 23.5; 23.129.

[35] Diodorus Siculus, *Library* 15.19.4.

[36] Plutarch, *Life of Agesilaus* 35.3.

[37] Diodorus Siculus, *Library* 15.50.5.

[38] Diodorus Siculus, *Library* 15.50.5.

[39] J. Roisman, 'Klearchos in Xenophon's Anabasis', *Scripta Classica Israelica*, 8/9, 1985–1989, 50.

[40] Xenophon, *Anabasis* 2.6.6.

negative behaviour or at least detrimental to his standing—this is clearly not the case with Clearchus. Ultimately, *philopolemos* does not offer any pathological instruction. It is a rather vague description offered by one source, during a long defence of the Spartan's actions, which does not offer it in any form of medical or behavioural exposition.

This issue of terminology is exacerbated by another adjective Xenophon uses to describe Clearchus, *philokindynos* (lover of danger/risk). Unlike *philopolemos*, *philokindynos* offers more potential to explain a specific set of potentially symptomatic behavioural traits. It explains his fondness to always lead the attack, and why he becomes visibly happy in times of real peril and danger.[41] This, surely, is a better example for Clearchus' addiction to the 'high' of combat, not least because it seems counterintuitive and therefore potentially symptomatic of an atypical response to war. Yet, Xenophon uses the word in two of his other works to suggest that being *philokyndynos* was a very desirable trait:

> What he proposed was as follows: to the private soldier, that he show himself obedient to the officers, ready for hardship, eager for danger but subject to good discipline, familiar with the duties required of a soldier.[42]

This usage by Xenophon suggests that Clearchus was not only a lover of risk, but that such a trait was a positive attribute in a commander. The term is also used by Plutarch to describe such men as Pericles and Alcibiades, and by the orator Isocrates to describe Heracles, no less.[43] So this term does not suggest a negative default in meaning. The only way this could be aligned with PTSD would be if it could be proven to be detrimental behaviour in the civic setting, but there is no example of this. Similarly, to suggest that Clearchus refused to return to Sparta because he was addicted to war and danger, conveniently leaves out the fact that numerous Spartan commanders resisted returning to Sparta when they were commissioned abroad.

[41] Xenophon, *Anabasis* 2.6.7, 10.

[42] Xenophon, *Cyropaedia* 2.1.22 (Translator Walter Miller, 1914). He repeats this sentiment in his *Hellenica*, 6.1.6.

[43] Pericles: Plutarch, *Life of Pericles* 7.1. Alcibiades: Plutarch, *Life of Alcibiades* 18.1. Heracles: Isocrates, *Helen* 10.17.

Cultural Aspects of Studies on the Presence of PTSD in the Past

It seems that recent scholarship is aware of the many methodological issues that have been raised in this chapter. Work on ancient PTSD, by historians in particular, will often contain a qualifying statement to the effect that cultural differences between past and present make it impossible to impose such a diagnosis on the past; and yet, they continue to use the model as a way to examine the texts.[44] However, we know that cultural factors underpin the definitions of mental illnesses and diagnoses.[45] We also know that cultural contexts determine the way those diagnoses are talked about and described in the source material.[46] This is before we acknowledge the fact that cultures often represent stereotypical behaviour as a means to validate their own observations.

If we consider modern-day media, generic mental illnesses have often been portrayed with stereotypical hallmarks of 'madness', such as the hearing of voices, repetitive movements such as rocking, and involuntary spasms such as a facial tic.[47] Another cultural factor we must consider is what the ancient Greeks, or Assyrians, or whichever culture, expected to

[44] S.S. Monoson, 'Socrates in Combat: Trauma and Resilience in Plato's Political Theory', in P. Meineck and D. Konstan (eds), *Combat Trauma and the Ancient Greeks* (New York: Palgrave Macmillan, 2014), p. 134; B. Steinbock 'Sufferings Too Great for Tears: The Destruction of the Athenian Expeditionary Corps in Sicily', in Melanie Jonasch (ed), *The Fight for Greek Sicily Society, Politics, and Landscape* (Oxford: Oxbow Books, 2020), pp. 76–8.

[45] Renato D. Alarcón, 'Culture, Cultural Factors and Psychiatric Diagnosis: Review and Projections' *World Psychiatry* 8, 2009, 131–39; Andrew Roderick Gilmoor, Adithy Adithy, and Barbara Regeer, 'The Cross-Cultural Validity of Post-traumatic Stress Disorder and Post-traumatic Stress Symptoms in the Indian Context: A Systematic Search and Review' *Frontiers in Psychiatry* 10.439, 2019; Guerda Nicolas, Anna Wheatley, and Casta Guillaume, 'Does One Trauma Fit All? Exploring the Relevance of PTSD Across Cultures', *International Journal of Culture and Mental Health* 8, 2015, 34–45.

[46] The best discussions of this methodological issue are found in 'Thinking About Mental Disorders in Classical Antiquity', in William V. Harris (ed), *Mental Disorders in the Classical World* (Leiden: Brill, 2013), and C. Thumiger and P.N. Singer, 'Introduction: Disease Classification and Mental Illness: Ancient and Modern Perspectives', in C. Thumiger and P.N. Singer (eds), *Mental Illness in Ancient Medicine: From Celsus to Paul of Aegina* (Leiden: Brill, 2018), 1–32.

[47] Or, as Otto Wahl observed, the common default is to portray a caricatured form of schizophrenia—Otto Wahl, *Media Madness: Public Images of Mental Illness* (New Brunswick: Rutgers University Press, 1995/2003), pp. 89–90.

see when they encountered insanity or madness. In the modern European medical model, we expect issues associated with the mind itself, such as delusions and hallucinations. The Greeks often portrayed forms of mania in very different ways. Commonly, we see a focus on the face, and in particular the eyes, as the most relevant depiction of an altered mental state, as is the presence of limb spasms and convulsions. In fact, many of the symptoms associated with the sacred disease, epilepsy, are 'included among the signs of mental suffering generally'.[48]

But more than this, culture determines how these symptoms, experiences, and behaviours are defined. If we discover PTSD-like symptoms that are not medicalised, that tells us something, and yet our attempt to medicalise them removes important cultural data inherent in the textual narrative. In fact, we are enforcing our own narrow cultural view on these symptoms as indicative of mental disorder onto cultures that do not share our interpretations. While our own medical tradition demands a categorised diagnosis, with a controlled list of symptoms, it is noted that this general model is often hard to utilise in practice, especially as the therapist or psychiatrist learns more about the individual patient.[49]

Mental illness categories have been formulated in the American-European cultural sphere, and diagnosis can often reflect ethno-cultural variances as much as an accurate reflection of symptoms.[50] Such an approach creates two problems: (1) we are inclined to dismiss other cultures' explanations for the same phenomena: (2) we prioritise our own cultural factors over others. The predominant factor discussed in the ancient PTSD debate is the act of killing and the exposure to death, something Crowley's work specifically targets to assert the relativist position.[51] But we are also missing other cultural imperatives that determine trauma,

[48] C. Thumiger, *A History of the Mind and Mental Health in Classical Greek Medical Thought* (Cambridge: Cambridge University Press, 2017), p. 48.

[49] B. Simon, '"Carving Nature at the Joints": The Dream of a Perfect Classification of Mental Illness', in William V. Harris (ed), *Mental Disorders in the Classical World* (Leiden: Brill, 2013), p. 37.

[50] S. Minsky, W. Vega, T. Miskimen, M. Gara, and J. Escobar, 'Diagnostic Patterns in Latino, African American, and European American Psychiatric Patients', *Arch Gen Psychiatry* 60.6, 2003, 637–44.

[51] Jason Crowley, 'Beyond the Universal Soldier: Combat Trauma in Classical Antiquity', in P. Meineck and D. Konstan (eds), *Combat Trauma and the Ancient Greeks* (New York: Palgrave Macmillan, 2014), pp. 111–12.

as well as different factors which we do not share and do not on their own suggest to us a symptomology of PTSD.

The universalist model of ancient PTSD relies on a neurobiological underpinning to PTSD being present in all humans, regardless of cultural or ethnic diversity. In such a model, the cultural factors in medicine and indeed in some symptom variation can be reconciled, because the underlying biological cause of PTSD and its major symptoms are universally present in all humans. Yet, the growing field of cultural neuroscience is bringing such a view into question. As Liddell and Johnson highlight in their review article on the field and its insight into PTSD studies: 'An expanding evidence base challenges the pervasive assumption that basic cognitive, perceptual, behavioural, and emotional processes are governed by neural systems that function universally in all humans'.[52] Cultural factors have been found to impact even the most innate and primal of autonomic human reactions, namely fear. We are not talking about the descriptions of fear, or how a culture considers 'fear', but things pertaining to the neurocircuitry of fear processing. Studies have found intercultural differences in physiological arousal responses, and even variances in amygdala responsivity.[53] In essence, new research is beginning to show that cultural factors can influence and shape automatic emotional and perception processes. These processes have until recently been considered universal and fixed, giving credence to a one-size-fits-all approach to PTSD and, in turn, giving validity to its use as a retrospective diagnosis.

When we consider the historical agent, we must acknowledge our limitations. Scouring the source material for symptoms is not the same as in-person diagnosis by a trained professional. In the very act of trying

[52] B. Liddell and L. Jobson, 'The Impact of Cultural Differences in Self-representation on the Neural Substrates of Posttraumatic Stress Disorder', *European Journal of Psychotraumatology* 7:1, 2016, 1–13, https://doi.org/10.3402/ejpt.v7.30464, accessed 22 December 21.

[53] Arousal response: K.G. Martinez, J.A. Franco-Chaves, M.R. Milad, and G.J. Quirk, 'Ethnic Differences in Physiological Responses to Fear Conditioned Stimuli', *PLoS One* 9, 12, 2014, e114977, http://dx.doi.org/10.1371/journal.pone.0114977, accessed 22 December 21.

Amygdala: B. Derntl, U. Habel, S. Robinson, C. Windischberger, I. Kryspin-Exner, R.C. Gur, and E. Moser, 'Culture But Not Gender Modulates Amygdala Activation During Explicit Emotion Recognition', *BMC Neuroscience* 13, 2011, 54; J.Y. Chiao, T. Iidaka, H.L. Gordon, J. Nogawa, M. Bar, E. Aminoff, N. Sadato, and N. Ambady, 'Cultural Specificity in Amygdala Response to Fear Faces', *Journal of Cognitive Neuroscience* 20.12, 2008, 2167–74.

to retrospectively diagnose a historic figure, we are breaking the so-called *Goldwater Rule*.[54] We must accept that any trauma or emotional processing is culturally reflective, not only in the symptomology, or lack thereof, but also in the very way the individual would have experienced the event and been received by society afterwards. We can no longer take for granted a basic principle of shared neurocircuitry, and must accept that the diagnosis of PTSD is not applicable to the ancient world.

Conclusions

Studies into ancient PTSD have, from the beginning, avoided a reliance on the clinical definition of the diagnosis. Such an admission shows, first and foremost, that the model of PTSD is not suitable for historic usage. This chapter has argued that such a methodological slant has encouraged researchers to cherry-pick symptoms from the diagnosis to suit the research agenda of the scholarship and has, as a result, under-represented the societal context of the evidence base.

The original studies identified a phenomenon in the source material, namely the psychological and behavioural impact of war on the individual. But the emphasis to align this with PTSD has resulted in a pervasive presentism in the analysis which undermines the potential to examine different cultural reactions, and different individual experiences of that phenomenon. This presentism is also highly problematic due to the ethno-cultural foundation of the modern diagnostic environment. As new research begins to explore the role of culture on even the most autonomic of human reactions, it is time for historians to allow the sources to speak for their own cultural interpretations and then examine the human experience within that framework.

Acknowledgements My thanks to my fellow editors for their feedback on this chapter, and also to Dr Jo Edge who read an earlier draft and gave me invaluable comments.

[54] American Psychological Association, *Principles of Medical Ethics with Annotations Especially Applicable to Psychiatry* (2013 edition), 7.3: 'it is unethical for a psychiatrist to offer a professional opinion unless he or she has conducted an examination and has been granted proper authorization for such a statement.'

Bibliography

Abdul-Hamid, Walid Khalid, and Jamie Hacker Hughes, 'Nothing New under the Sun: Post-traumatic Stress Disorders in the Ancient World', *Early Science and Medicine* 19.6, 2014, 549–57.

Ackerknecht, Erwin H., 'Psychopathology, Primitive Medicine and Primitive Culture', *Bulletin of the History of Medicine* 14, 1943, 30–67.

Alarcón, Renato D., 'Culture, Cultural Factors and Psychiatric Diagnosis: Review and Projections', *World Psychiatry* 8, 2009, 131–39.

American Psychological Association, *Principles of Medical Ethics with Annotations Especially Applicable to Psychiatry* (2013 edition), 7.3.

American Psychiatric Association, *Diagnostics and Statistical Manual of Mental Disorders-5* (Washington: American Psychiatric Association, 2019).

Arrizabalaga, J., 'Problematizing Retrospective Diagnosis in the History of Disease', *Asclepio* 54, 2002, 51–70.

Baker, Dana Lee, *The Politics of Neurodiversity: Why Public Policy Matters* (Boulder: Lynne Reiner, 2011).

Bark, N.M. 'On the History of Schizophrenia: Evidence of Its Existence Before 1800', *New York State Journal of Medicine* 88.7, 1988, 374–83.

Berrios, G.E., 'Classifications in Psychiatry: A Conceptual History', *Australian and New Zealand Journal of Psychiatry* 33.2, 1999, 145–60.

Bracken, P.J., 'Post-modernity and Post-traumatic Stress Disorder', *Social Science & Medicine* 53.6, 2001, 733–43.

Chiao, J.Y., T. Iidaka, H.L. Gordon, J. Nogawa, M. Bar, E. Aminoff, N. Sadato, and N. Ambady, 'Cultural Specificity in Amygdala Response to Fear Faces', *Journal of Cognitive Neuroscience* 20.12, 2008, 2167–74.

Crowley, Jason, 'Beyond the Universal Soldier: Combat Trauma in Classical Antiquity', in P. Meineck and D. Konstan (eds), *Combat Trauma and the Ancient Greeks* (New York: Palgrave Macmillan, 2014), 105–30.

Cunningham, A., 'Identifying Disease in the Past: Cutting the Gordian Knot', *Asclepio* 54, 2002, 13–34.

DePoy, E., and S.F. Gilson, *Studying Disability: Multiple Theories and Responses* (London: Sage, 2011).

Derntl, B., U. Habel, S. Robinson, C. Windischberger, I. Kryspin-Exner, R.C. Gur, and E. Moser, 'Culture But Not Gender Modulates Amygdala Activation During Explicit Emotion Recognition', *BMC Neuroscience* 13, 2011, 54. https://doi.org/10.1186/1471-2202-13-54

Fraguas, D., 'Problems with Retrospective Studies of the Presence of Schizophrenia', *History of Psychiatry* 20.1, 2009, 61–71.

Gilmoor, Andrew Roderick, Adithy Adithy, and Barbara Regeer, 'The Cross-Cultural Validity of Post-traumatic Stress Disorder and Post-traumatic Stress Symptoms in the Indian Context: A Systematic Search and Review', *Frontiers in Psychiatry* 10.439, 2019, 1–24.

Haldipur, C.V., 'Madness in Ancient India: Concept of Insanity in Charaka Samhita (1st century A.D.)', *Comprehensive Psychiatry* 25.3, 1984, 335–44.

Harris, W.V., 'Thinking About Mental Disorders in Classical Antiquity', in William V. Harris (ed), *Mental Disorders in the Classical World* (Leiden: Brill, 2013), 1–23,

Jeste, D.V., R. del Carmen, J.B. Lohr, and R.J. Wyatt, 'Did Schizophrenia Exist Before the Eighteenth Century?' *Comprehensive Psychiatry* 26.6, 1985, 493–503.

Jones, Edgar, and Simon Wessely, 'War Syndromes: The Impact of Culture on Medically Unexplained Symptoms', *Medical History* 49, 2005, 55–78.

Karenberg, A., and F.P. Moog, 'Next Emperor Please! No End to Retrospective Diagnosis', *Journal of the History of the Neurosciences* 13.2, 2004, 143–49.

Kirmayer, L.J., 'Confusion of the Senses: Implications of Ethnocultural Variations in Somatoform and Dissociative Disorders for PTSD', in A.J. Marsella, M.J. Friedman, E.T. Gerrity, and R.M. Scurfield (eds), *Ethnocultural Aspects of Posttraumatic Stress Disorder: Issues, Research, and Clinical Applications* (Washington, DC: American Psychological Association, 1996), pp. 131–63.

Leven, K.H., '"At Times These Ancient Facts Seem to Lie Before Me Like a Patient on a Hospital Bed"—Retrospective Diagnosis and Ancient Medical History,' in Manfred Horstmanshoff and Marten Stol (eds), *Magic and Rationality in Ancient Near Eastern and Graeco-Roman Medicine* (Leiden: Brill, 2004), pp. 369–86.

Liddell, B., and L. Jobson, 'The Impact of Cultural Differences in Self-representation on the Neural Substrates of Posttraumatic Stress Disorder', *European Journal of Psychotraumatology* 7.1, 2016, 30464. https://doi.org/10.3402/ejpt.v7.30464, accessed 22 December 21.

Martinez, K.G., J.A. Franco-Chaves, M.R. Milad, and G.J. Quirk, 'Ethnic Differences in Physiological Responses to Fear Conditioned Stimuli', *PLoS One* 9,12, 2014, e114977. https://doi.org/10.1371/journal.pone.0114977, accessed 22 December 21.

Metzge, N., 'Railway Spine, Shell-shock and Psychological Trauma: The Limits of Retrospetcive Diagnosis', in Eve-Marie Becker, Jan Dochhorn, Else Holt (eds), *Trauma and Traumatization in Individual and Collective Dimensions: Insights from Biblical Studies and Beyond* (Gottingen: Vandenhoek & Ruprecht GmBH, 2014), pp. 43–61.

Minsky, S., W. Vega, T. Miskimen, M. Gara, and J. Escobar, 'Diagnostic Patterns in Latino, African American, and European American Psychiatric Patients', *Arch Gen Psychiatry* 60.6, 2003, 637–44.

Monoson, S.S., 'Socrates in Combat: Trauma and Resilience in Plato's Political Theory', in P. Meineck and D. Konstan (eds), *Combat Trauma and the Ancient Greeks* (New York: Palgrave Macmillan, 2014), pp. 131–62.

Nicolas, Guerda, Anna Wheatley, and Casta Guillaume, 'Does One Trauma Fit All? Exploring the Relevance of PTSD Across Cultures', *International Journal of Culture and Mental Health* 8, 2015, 34–45.

O'Brien, S., *Traumatic Events and Mental Health* (Cambridge: Cambridge University Press, 1998).

Otsuka, K., and Sakai, A., 'Haizmann's Madness: The Concept of Bizarreness and the Diagnosis of Schizophrenia', *History of Psychiatry* 15.1, 2004, 73–82.

Rees, O., 'We Need to Talk About Epizelus: PTSD and the Ancient World', *Medical Humanities* 46.1, 2020, 46–54.

Roisman, J., 'Klearchos in Xenophon's Anabasis', *Scripta Classica Israelica*, 8–9, 1985–1989, 30–52.

Scurlock, J., and Burton Anderson, *Diagnoses in Assyrian and Babylonian Medicine* (Chicago: University of Illinois Press, 2005).

Shay, J., *Achilles in Vietnam: Trauma and the Undoing of Character* (New York: Athenaeum, 1994).

Shay, J., 'Moral Injury', *Intertexts* 16.1, 2012, 57–66.

Simon, B., '"Carving Nature at the Joints": The Dream of a Perfect Classification of Mental Illness', in William V. Harris (ed), *Mental Disorders in the Classical World* (Leiden: Brill, 2013), 27–40.

Steinbock, B. 'Sufferings Too Great for Tears': The Destruction of the Athenian Expeditionary Corps in Sicily', in Melanie Jonasch (ed), *The Fight for Greek Sicily Society, Politics, and Landscape* (Oxford: Oxbow Books, 2020), pp. 73–98.

Stone, M.H. *Healing the Mind: A History of Psychiatry from Antiquity to the Present* (New York: W. W. Norton, 1997).

Thumiger, C., 'The Early Greek Medical Vocabulary of Insanity', in William V. Harris (ed), *Mental Disorders in the Classical World* (Leiden: Brill, 2013), pp. 61–95.

Thumiger, C., *A History of the Mind and Mental Health in Classical Greek Medical Thought* (Cambridge: Cambridge University Press, 2017).

Thumiger, C., and P.N. Singer, 'Introduction. Disease Classification and Mental Illness: Ancient and Modern Perspectives', in C. Thumiger and P.N. Singer (eds), *Mental Illness in Ancient Medicine: From Celsus to Paul of Aegina* (Leiden: Brill, 2018), pp. 1–32.

Tritle, L., *Melos to My Lai* (London: Routledge, 2000).

Wahl, Otto, *Media Madness: Public Images of Mental Illness* (New Brunswick: Rutgers University Press, 1995/2003).

Young, A., *The Harmony of Illusions* (Princeton: Princeton University Press, 1995).

Youssef, H.A., and F.A. Youssef, 'Evidence for the Existence of Schizophrenia in Medieval Islamic Society', *History of Psychiatry* 7, 1996, 55–62.

A Collective War Trauma in Classical Athens? Coping with the Human Cost of Warfare in Aeschylus' *Persians*

Giorgia Proietti

War Trauma Between Psychology and History—Ancient and Modern

As both a historical phenomenon and a historiographical category, war trauma was born in the twentieth century. It entered the field of military psychopathology in the aftermath of First World War, and was first classified as a type of Post-Traumatic Stress Disorder (PTSD) after the Vietnam War; today, as a consequence of the massive military engagement of the Western world in the Middle East, it has become an urgent issue of public interest especially in the USA, and also, though with a comparatively minor incidence, in the UK and elsewhere in Europe.[1] Known

[1] M.A. Crocq and L. Crocq, 'From Shell Shock and War Neurosis to Posttraumatic Stress Disorder: A History of Psychotraumatology', *Dialogues in Clinical Neurosciences* 2.1, 2000, 47–55; B. Shephard, *A War of Nerves. Soldiers and Psychiatrists in the Twentieth Century* (Cambridge, MA: Harvard University Press, 2001).

G. Proietti (✉)
University of Trento, Trento, Italy
e-mail: giorgia.proietti@unitn.it

O. Rees et al. (eds.), *Combat Stress in Pre-modern Europe*, Mental Health in Historical Perspective,
https://doi.org/10.1007/978-3-031-09947-2_3

also as war neurosis, it refers to the veterans' difficulties in both coping with feelings and situations they had experienced during war, and recovering their normal lives as civilians afterwards. The medical treatment of veterans' war trauma in the USA provided the chance for an interdisciplinary encounter with Classics: starting from the 90s, the American psychiatrist Jonathan Shay successfully introduced Homer into his therapy of combat stress. Veterans were in fact able to pinpoint symptoms of their post-traumatic syndrome in the behaviour of several protagonists within ancient Greek literature, and therapeutically identify themselves with them.[2] Despite the serious methodological risks implicated in this approach, which takes for granted the universality of war trauma in totally different historical contexts,[3] the dialogue concerning this phenomenon

[2] J. Shay, *Achilles in Vietnam: Combat Trauma and the Undoing of Character* (New York: Atheneum, 1995); J. Shay, *Odysseus in America. Combat Trauma and the Trials of Homecoming* (New York: Scribner, 2002); J. Shay, 'Homer's Leaders in America's Forces: Leadership and Prevention of Psychological and Moral Injury', in M. Cosmopoulos (ed), *Experiencing War. Trauma and Society from Ancient Greece to the Iraq War* (Chicago: Ares, 2007), pp. 258–77. Soon afterwards, other scholars further developed the connection between ancient and modern war trauma, and purportedly pinpointed symptoms of today's veterans' war trauma in the behaviour of several characters within Greek literature (both epic and tragedy) and history: psychological conditions such as Achilles' wrath, Philoctetes' suicidal will, Epizelus' blindness, Clearchus' belligerence, Alexander the Great's madness or Alexander's army's mutiny—just to name a few instances—are thought to be the alleged precedents to modern combat-induced PTSD. Especially notable in this regard is the work by L.A. Tritle, *From Melos to My Lai. War and Survival* (London: Routledge, 2000); 'Alexander and the Killing of Cleitus the Black', in W. Heckel and L.A. Tritle (eds), *Crossroads of History: The Age of Alexander* (Claremont: Regina Books, 2003), pp. 127–46; 'Xenophon's Portrait of Clearchus. A Study in Post-Traumatic Stress Disorder', in C. Tuplin (ed), *Xenophon and his World* (Stuttgart: Franz Steiner Verlag, 2004), pp. 325–39; 'Gorgias, the Encomium of Helen, and the Trauma of War', *Clio's Psyche* 16.2, 2009, 195–99; ''Ravished Minds' in the Ancient World', in P. Meineck and D. Konstan (eds), *Combat Trauma and the Ancient Greeks* (New York: Palgrave, 2014), pp. 87–103.

[3] In addition to the fact that we do not have at our disposal anything comparable to the personal writings or the medical records of World War I and World War II soldiers, or the oral reports of modern veterans, on the one hand the analysis of the cultural, social, environmental, and tactical factors characterizing war in ancient Greece questions the hoplites' exposure to PTSD (J. Crowley, *The Psychology of the Athenian Hoplite. The Culture of Combat in Classical Athens* (Cambridge: Cambridge University Press, 2012) and 'Beyond the Universal Soldier: Combat Trauma in Classical Antiquity', in Meineck and Konstan, *Combat Trauma*, pp. 105–30), on the other hand the analysis of the relationship between the *oikos* and the polis, as well as of the transition of the hoplites from domestic and military service and vice versa challenges the universalist model and

between ancient and modern times has proven its potential: theatre for veterans (for instance, the *Theatre of War* by Brian Doerries; the *Ancient Greeks/Modern Lives* as well as the *Warrior Chorus* project by Peter Meineck's Aquila Theatre) has recently shown how Greek tragedy today can help veterans and their families affected by combat stress, by triggering a cathartic mechanism which is analogue to the ancient one, as it is described by Aristotle.[4]

Apart from the study of war-induced PTSD, the Holocaust was the decisive turning point in the historical development of modern theories on trauma as it is currently explored, not only in psychological but also in social, cultural, and historical terms.[5] In that respect, the term 'trauma' refers not only to individual traumas, i.e. to Holocaust survivors' difficulty to cope with memories of what they suffered and recover their normal life afterwards, but also to the mechanisms according to which trauma

demands for a historical contextualization (O. Rees, *Military Departures, Homecomings and Death in Classical Athens. Hoplite Transitions* (London: Bloomsbury, 2022). For a survey of the current approaches, with methodological problems and further literature, see G. Proietti, 'Can an Ancient Truth become an Old Lie? A Few Methodological Remarks Concerning Current Comparative Research on War and its Aftermath', in M. Giangiulio, E. Franchi and G. Proietti (eds), *Commemorating War and War Dead. Ancient and Modern* (Stuttgart: Franz Steiner Verlag, 2019), pp. 80–85; B. Steinbock, 'Sufferings too Great for Tears. The Destruction of the Athenian Expeditionary Corps in Sicily', in M. Jonasch (ed.), *The Fight for Greek Sicily. Society, Politics, and Landscape* (Oxford: Oxbow Books, 2020), pp. 73–81. That does not mean we must quit wondering about PTSD in relation to war in antiquity, O. Rees, 'We Need to Talk about Epizelus: 'PTSD' and the Ancient World', *Medical Humanities*, 46.1, 2019, 46–54.

[4] P. Meineck, 'Combat Trauma and the Tragic Stage: 'Restoration' by Cultural Catharsis', *Intertexts* 16.1, 2012, 7–24; B. Doerries, B., *Theatre of War. What Ancient Greek Tragedies Can Teach Us Today* (New York: Scribe, 2015).

[5] See e.g. M. Hirsch and L. Spitzer, 'The Witness in the Archive: Holocaust Studies/Memory Studies', in S. Radstone and B. Schwarz (eds), *Memory. Histories, Theories, Debates* (New York: Fordham University Press, 2010), pp. 390–405; J. Brunner and N. Zajde, *Holocaust und Trauma: kritische Perspektiven zur Entstehung und Wirkung eines Paradigmas* (Göttingen: Wallstein, 2011). The Holocaust is a perfect example of a two-sided collective trauma, which in different ways and with different meanings crystallized in both the victims' and the perpetrators' collective memory and identity. Several studies which sophistically engage with trauma from a theoretical standpoint extensively refer to the Holocaust as the event which epitomizes historical trauma (e.g. D. La Capra, *Writing History, Writing Trauma* (Baltimore-London: John Hopkins University Press, 2001); J.C. Alexander, *Trauma. A Social Theory* (Cambridge; Cambridge University Press, 2012); G. Hirschberger, 'Collective Trauma and the Social Construction of Meaning', *Frontiers in Psychology* 9, 2018, 1–18.

develops, roots, and perpetuates, generation after generation, in a group's collective memory, until it becomes a component of their cultural identity: in other words, it becomes a 'collective trauma'. As psychologist Gilad Hirschberger has recently defined it:

> The term collective trauma refers to the psychological reactions to a traumatic event that affect an entire society; it does not merely reflect an historical fact, the recollection of a terrible event that happened to a group of people. It suggests that the tragedy is represented in the collective memory of the group, and like all forms of memory it comprises not only a reproduction of the events, but also an ongoing reconstruction of the trauma in an attempt to make sense of it. Collective memory of trauma is different from individual memory because collective memory persists beyond the lives of the direct survivors of the events, and is remembered by group members that may be far removed from the traumatic events in time and space.[6]

Since then, trauma studies have gradually become integrated into contemporary history and culture, and the notion of 'collective trauma' (or 'cultural trauma') has become more and more frequent in historical research, in reference to groups which in any time and place in history have collectively experienced a high-impacting event, which they have socially constructed and transmitted as a collective trauma.[7] Most recently, also in the field of ancient history, the strictly psychological approach to war

[6] Hirschberger, 'Collective Trauma', 1. Together with 'collective trauma', an analogue current expression is that of 'cultural trauma' (Alexander, J.C. et al. *Cultural Trauma and Collective Identity* (Berkeley: University of California Press 2004); Alexander, *Trauma*). Holocaust is also among the most notable and more studied examples of transgenerational transmission of trauma (or secondary traumatization): see e.g. N. Kellermann, 'Transmitted Holocaust Trauma: Curse or Legacy? The Aggravating and Mitigating Factors of Holocaust Transmission', *The Israel Journal of Psychiatry and Related Science* 45, 2008, 263–71, with previous literature.

[7] Within an extensive literature, for a general view on trauma and history, with a special focus on memory and identity related questions, see for instance C. Cathy, *Trauma: Explorations in Memory* (Baltimore: John Hopkins University Press, 1995); C. Cathy, *Unclaimed Experience: Trauma, Narrative and History* (Baltimore: John Hopkins University Press, 1996); R. Leys, *Trauma. A Genealogy* (Chicago: Chicago University Press, 2000); R. Luckhurst, *The Trauma Question* (London: Routledge, 2008); N. Hunt, *Memory, War and Trauma* (Cambridge: Cambridge University Press, 2010). For collective trauma as a social construction, having to do more with social understanding and

trauma has been paired by a broad interest into the '*revers de la guerre*' (from Payen's recent book title), i.e. the traumatic consequences of war on entire groups and communities, including both veterans and civilians, and the coping mechanisms they elaborate to face harmful events such as the destruction of their city, mass enslavement, or a high number of casualties.[8] The latter theme figures prominently in Aeschylus' *Persians*.

Aeschylus' *Persians* in Post-War Athens

In 472 BC, the *Persians* presented the Persians' defeat at Salamis. The choice of this topic has been variously interpreted. According to the two main views, both implying a political reading of the play, Aeschylus' aim was either to relish the enemy's sufferings and glorify the Greek (mostly Athenian) recent victory, or to warn the Athenians against the danger of imperialism.[9] While both of these interpretations might at the same time

the attribution of meanings, than with the intrinsic nature of the events themselves, see Alexander, *Trauma*; Hirschberger, 'Collective Trauma'.

[8] P. Payen, *Les revers de la guerre en Grèce ancienne: histoire et historiographie* (Paris: Belin, 2012); K.A. Raaflaub, '*Lysistrata* and War's Impact on the Home Front', in V. Caston and S.-M. Weineck (eds), *Our Ancient Wars. Rethinking War through the Classics* (Ann Arbor: University of Michigan Press, 2016), pp. 38–74; K.A. Raaflaub, 'War and the City: The Brutality of War and its Impact on the Community', in Meineck and Konstan (eds), *Combat Trauma*, pp. 15–46; C. Bearzot, 'Le conseguenze della guerra nell'antichità', *Studium* 111, 2015, 95–106; R. Garland, *Athens Burning. The Persian Invasion of Greece and the Evacuation of Attica* (Baltimore: John Hopkins University Press, 2016); P. Meineck, 'Thebes as High-Collateral-Damage Target. Moral Accountability for Killing in Aeschylus' *Seven against Thebes*', in I. Torrance (ed), *Aeschylus and War: Comparative Perspectives on* Seven against Thebes (Abingdon, Oxon: Routledge, 2017), pp. 49–70; G. Proietti, 'Fare i conti con la guerra. Forme del discorso civico ad Atene nel V secolo', in E. Franchi and G. Proietti (eds), *Conflict in Communities. Forward-looking Memories in Classical Athens* (Trento: Trento University Press, 2017), pp. 69–108; Torrance (ed), *Aeschylus and War*, 2017. An overview of the current diversified approaches to war trauma (individual and collective, psychological and historical) in ancient Greek history is offered by the volumes edited by M. Cosmopoulos (ed), *Experiencing War. Trauma and Society from Ancient Greece to the Iraq War* (Chicago Ill: Ares, 2007); Meineck and Konstan, *Combat Trauma*; Caston V. and S.-M. Weineck (eds), *Our Ancient Wars:* Rethinking *War through the Classics* (Ann Arbor: University of Michigan Press, 2016); Torrance (ed), *Aeschylus and War*, 2017.

[9] Within these major trends, the extensive bibliography concerned with a political reading of the *Persians* is significantly diversified and cannot be reviewed here; see most notably E. Hall, *Inventing the Barbarian: Greek Self-Definition Through Tragedy* (Oxford: Clarendon Press, 1989); E. Hall (ed), *Aeschylus. Persians* (Warminster: Aris and Phillips,

be true, I find difficulties with relating the alleged political goal (be it the patriotic celebration of or the admonition to Athens) to the general function of a drama—that is, leading the civic community first to identify themselves with, and then to alienate themselves from, the situation on the stage, in order to reach the tragic catharsis, in Aristotle's terms.[10] In other terms, in the two current interpretations, I cannot comprehend the tragic mechanism which connects the representation of the enemy's defeat with the delivery of a specific political message, whatever it was, and the cathartic process proper of every drama, and I am even less prone to accept one function at the price of excluding the other.[11]

I suggest therefore changing perspective and taking into account a third possible interpretation—which can co-exist with the other two—of Aeschylus' choice of the subject and its function. In other terms, I think we should try to place the *Persians* in context, and relate the content of the play to the horizon of collective memories, emotions, and expectations of the Athenian civic community in the aftermath of

1996); C. Pelling, 'Aeschylus' *Persae* and History', in C. Pelling (ed), *Greek Tragedy and the Historian* (Oxford: Clarendon Press, 1997), pp. 1–19; T. Harrison, *The Emptiness of Asia. Aeschylus'* Persians *and the History of the Fifth Century* (London: Bloomsbury, 2000), pp. 103–15; D. Rosenbloom (ed), *Aeschylus. Persians* (London: Duckworth, 2006), pp. 141–46; A.F. Garvie (ed), *Aeschylus'* Persae, *with Introduction and Commentary* (Oxford: Oxford University Press, 2009), pp. xvi–xxii. A recent survey of the political readings of the play is in T. Lockwood, 'The Political Theorizing of Aeschylus' *Persians*', *Interpretations* 43, 2017, 383–401.

[10] According to Aristotle, the catharsis is the outcome of a double process, one homeopathic (identification → terror), the other allopathic (detachment → pity): cf. *Poetics*, 1449b, 20ff; *Rhetoric*, II 1382a (on terror); 1385b (on pity). Cf. also *Politica*, 1342a 5ff. See Woodruff in H.M. Roisman (ed), *The Encyclopedia of Greek Tragedy* (Oxford: Oxford University Press, 2014), *s.v.* 'Aristotle and Greek Tragedy (Purpose of)', with an outline of the debate surrounding the interpretation of Aristotle's theory, and main literature.

[11] Ronsenbloom, *Aeschylus*: *Persians*, p. 11: 'The central interpretative problem of the play is whether it is a tragedy in the canonical sense - an enactment that can arouse sympathetic emotions such as pity and fear in the audience - or a depiction of Persian defeat and lament that celebrates Greek military and cultural superiority, inducing *Schadenfreude* at the spectacle of the Persian pain', with wider discussion at pp. 141–45. On the *Persians* as a tragedy, see also Hall, *Aeschylus. Persians*, pp. 16–19; Garvie, *Aeschylus'* Persae, pp. xxii–xxxii; M. Hopman, 'Layered Stories in Aeschylus' *Persians*', in J. Grethlein and A. Rengakos (eds), *Narratology and Interpretation: The Content of Narrative Form in Ancient Literature* (Berlin-New York: Walter de Gruyter, 2009), pp. 357–76, although holding a different view than my own, also considers psychological issues concerning the Athenians' reactions to the play and makes a notable attempt to reconcile the contents of the play with the Aristotelian categories of fear and pity.

the Persian Wars. It is in my view widely overlooked that the play was represented in front of people who were fresh from a direct (in case of veterans) or indirect (in case of civilians) involvement in the war, and were also still involved in the ongoing war against the Persians in the Aegean Sea; in other terms, the play was represented in front of people who were deeply engaged in coping with the difficulties typical of a post-war period. When the *Persians* was on stage, Athens (and especially the Acropolis, just above the theatre of Dionysus) still exhibited the traces of the Persian destruction, and citizens were still toiling away at the reconstruction of the city infrastructures and, most of all, their houses.[12] Even more importantly, people attending the *Persians* included veterans of the battle of Salamis, and civilians, whose life had been profoundly changed as a consequence of the war: men who had been seriously injured or mutilated, women who had lost their husbands, parents who had lost their children, young men who had lost their fathers, and entire families who had been forced to leave their house and found it pillaged, if not destroyed. The context in which the *Persians* were staged therefore was not (or at least not only) that of a general excitement for the victory over the barbarians, as it is often stated, but that of a canonical post-war period, featuring dramatically urgent dynamics, from both a social and psychological standpoint.

Aeschylus' *Persians*: Coping with Unprecedented War Casualties

The theme of death in war, and that of the extensive sufferings as a result of war were at that time especially prominent. Beginning with the Persian wars, and all throughout the *Pentecontaetia*, the Athenian civic community had to cope with a massive military effort and, accordingly, unprecedented numbers of casualties: the dead, the wounded, the missing, and the ripples of grief and bereavement their fate generated back

[12] For post-Persian Athens, and especially the post-Persian Acropolis as a 'landscape of trauma', or 'site of trauma', see G. Proietti, 'Athens as a 'Landscape of Trauma': Phrynichus' *Sack of Miletus* and the Aftermath of the Persian Wars', in L. Cecchet, Ch. Degelmann and M. Patzelt (eds), *Impact of War on the Home Front in the Ancient World* (Cambridge: Cambridge University Press, 2019), pp. 79–98.

home.[13] If placed in this context, the representation of the Persian defeat at Salamis takes on a different colour: not only the political and military side of it, but also the psychological and emotional one was at the centre of the play. By focusing on the sufferings of the survivors, such as Xerxes, who pray for the fate of their beloved ones and mourn their death, the play represents the pain suffered by the Persians concerning the human cost of warfare.

What was the point of representing the enemy's sufferings? Certainly, the Athenians would not pity or empathize with those who were responsible for their own pain. I suggest that the pain of the Persians represented the pain of the Athenians,[14] who were therefore moved to empathy; at the same time, though, the adoption of the Persian perspective worked precisely as the requested 'filter', necessary to tragic catharsis, which

[13] On Athens' 'military hyperactivity' during the fifth century, see P. Hunt, 'Athenian Militarism and Recourse to War', in D. Pritchard (ed), *War, Democracy and Culture in Classical Athens* (Cambridge: Cambridge University Press, 2010), pp. 225–42; D.M. Pritchard, 'The Symbiosis between Democracy and War: The Case of Ancient Athens', in D.M. Pritchard (ed), *War, Democracy and Culture in Classical Athens* (Cambridge: Cambridge University Press, 2010), pp. 1–62. In the casualty list which refers to the fallen on six different battlefronts in 460/59 BC (*IG* I^3 1147), for instance, under the Erechtheid tribe by itself are listed 177 names.

[14] For the interpretation of the play as a vehicle for identification with the enemy around a shared experience of loss and death, see Hopman 'Layered Stories', with previous bibliography.

Phrynichus a few years earlier had missed when he put on scene the sack of Miletus.[15]

First of all, the identification between the Persians' and the Athenians' pain is suggested by two lists of dead Persians encapsulated in the play, which remind of the Athenian casualty lists. After the first lament of the chorus of elderly counsellors at the Persian court (ll. 256–89),[16] the messenger first announces the Persian defeat at Salamis, and then reassures the anxious Queen Atossa about the fate of Xerxes (ll. 290–301):[17]

[15] According to Herodotus 6.21.2, Phrynichus' play made the Athenians break into tears and ban any future reproduction of the play: the sack of Miletus reminded them, in fact, οἰκήια κακά (their own pains). In another article, I suggest that the play must be dated soon after the Persian sack of Athens (see also J. Roisman, 'On Phrynichos' *Sack of Miletus* and *Phoinissai*', *Eranos* 86, 1988, 15–23), and that, apart from the fact that the Athenians were understandably more sympathetic with the consanguineous Ionians than with the Persians (though the former had fought on the Persian side in the second Persian war), the Athenian reaction can be imputed to a revival of the sack of their own city, which was still at the core of a traumatic memory. See Proietti, 'Athens as a 'Landscape of Trauma'', with literature. On dramatic distance between the play world and that of the audience, and tragic indeterminancy (spatial and temporal) as essential features of tragedy, see P.E. Easterling, 'Anachronism in Greek Tragedy', *Journal of Hellenistic Studies*,1985, 105, 1–10; P.E. Easterling, 'Constructing the Heroic', in C.B.R. Pelling (ed), *Greek Tragedy and the Historian* (Oxford: Clarendon Press, 1997), pp. 21–37; W. Allan and A. Kelly, 'Listening to Many Voices: Greek Tragedy as Popular Art', in A. Marmodoro and J. Hill (eds), *The Author's Voice in Classical and Late Antiquity* (Oxford: Oxford University Press, 2013), pp. 99–101; C. Sourvinou-Inwood, *Tragedy and Athenian Religion* (Lanham MD.: Lexington Books, 2003); S. Mills, '*Ektos sumphoras*: Tragic Athens', *Polis* 34, 2017, 208–25, esp. 212–15; S. Mills, *Drama, Oratory and Thucydides in Fifth-Century Athens: Teaching Imperial Lessons* (London: Routledge, 2020), ch. 2, with further literature.

[16] The second lament of the chorus in the play is in ll. 908–1077 and is commented upon below.

[17] Texts and Translations of Aeschylus' *Persians* are from Alan H. Sommerstein (ed and trans), *Persians. Seven Against Thebes. Suppliants. Prometheus* (Cambridge, Mass.: Harvard University Press, 2008).

Ἄτοσσα σιγῶ πάλαι δύστηνος ἐκπεπληγμένη κακοῖς: ὑπερβάλλει γὰρ ἥδε συμφορὰ τὸ μήτε λέξαι μήτ' ἐρωτῆσαι πάθη. ὅμως δ' ἀνάγκη πημονὰς βροτοῖς φέρειν θεῶν διδόντων: πᾶν δ' ἀναπτύξας πάθος λέξον καταστάς, κεἰ στένεις κακοῖς ὅμως· τίς οὐ τέθνηκε, τίνα δὲ καὶ πενθήσομεν τῶν ἀρχελείων, ὅστ' ἐπὶ σκηπτουχίᾳ ταχθεὶς ἄνανδρον τάξιν ἠρήμου θανών;	**Atossa** I have been silent all this time because I was struck dumb with misery by this catastrophe. The event is so monstrous that one can neither speak nor ask about the sufferings it involved. Still, we mortals have no choice but to endure the sorrows the gods send us; so compose yourself and speak, revealing all that has happened, even if you are groaning under the weight of the disaster. Who has survived, and which of the leaders of the host must we mourn, who after being assigned to hold a staff of command perished and so left his post deserted and unmanned?
Ἄγγελος Ξέρξης μὲν αὐτὸς ζῇ τε καὶ φάος βλέπει.	**Messenger** Well, Xerxes himself is alive and sees the light of day.
Ἄτοσσα ἐμοῖς μὲν εἶπας δώμασιν φάος μέγα καὶ λευκὸν ἦμαρ νυκτὸς ἐκ μελαγχίμου.	**Queen** To my house at least your words come as a great relief, like bright day shining out after a pitch-dark night.

The messenger then makes a long list of Persian commanders who had lost their lives in battle (ll. 302–320):

Ἄγγελος
Ἀρτεμβάρης δὲ μυρίας ἵππου βραβεὺς
στύφλους παρ' ἀκτὰς θείνεται Σιληνιῶν·
χὠ χιλίαρχος Δαδάκης πληγῇ δορὸς
πήδημα κοῦφον ἐκ νεὼς ἀφήλατο·
Τενάγων τ' ἀριστεὺς Βακτρίων ἰθαιγενὴς
θαλασσόπληκτον νῆσον Αἴαντος πολεῖ
Λίλαιος, Ἀρσάμης τε κἀργήστης τρίτος,
οἵδ' ἀμφὶ νῆσον τὴν πελειοθρέμμονα
δινούμενοι 'κύρισσον ἰσχυρὰν χθόνα,
πηγαῖς τε Νείλου γειτονῶν Αἰγυπτίου
Φαρνοῦχος, οἵ τε ναὸς ἐκ μιᾶς πέσον
Ἀρκτεύς, Ἀδεύης, καὶ φερεσσάκης τρίτος,
ἵππου μελαίνης ἡγεμὼν τρισμυρίας.
Χρυσεὺς Μάταλλος μυριόνταρχος θανών,
πυρσὴν ζαπληθῆ δάσκιον γενειάδα
ἔτεγγ', ἀμείβων χρῶτα πορφυρέᾳ βαφῇ·
καὶ Μᾶγος Ἄραβος, Ἀρτάβης τε Βάκτριος,
σκληρᾶς μέτοικος γῆς, ἐκεῖ κατέφθιτο.
Ἄμιστρις Ἀμφιστρεύς τε πολύπονον δόρυ
νωμῶν, ὅ τ' ἐσθλὸς Ἀριόμαρδος ἄρδεσιν
πένθος παρασχών, Σεισάμης θ' ὁ Μύσιος,
Θάρυβίς τε πεντήκοντα πεντάκις νεῶν
ταγός, γένος Λυρναῖος, εὐειδὴς ἀνήρ,
κεῖται θανὼν δείλαιος οὐ μάλ' εὐτυχῶς·
Συέννεσίς τε πρῶτος εἰς εὐψυχίαν,
Κιλίκων ἄπαρχος, εἷς ἀνὴρ πλεῖστον πόνον
ἐχθροῖς παρασχών, εὐκλεῶς ἀπώλετο
τοσόνδ' ἐπαρχόντων ὑπεμνήσθην πέρι·
πολλῶν παρόντων δ' ὀλίγ' ἀπαγγέλλω κακά.

Messenger:
But Artambares, the commander of ten thousand horse, is being pounded against the rugged shores of Sileniae; Dadaces, commander of a thousand, was struck by a spear and took an effortless leap from his ship; and the excellent Tenagon, a noble of the Bactrians, now wanders around the wave-beaten island of Ajax. Lilaeus, Arsames, and Argestes - these three vanquished men were beating their heads against the hard rocks around the island where doves breed, as was Pharnuchus, whose home was near the stream of Egyptian Nile and three who fell from one ship, Arcteus, Adeues, and Pheresseues, leader of thirty thousand dark-skinned horsemen. Matallus of Chrysa, commander of ten thousand, perished; his fully, bushy, redish beard got a soaking, and a purple dye changed the colour of his skin. And Magus the Arab and Artabes the Bactrian, now a permanent resident in a harsh country, perished there too; and Amistris, and Amphistreus who wielded a spear that caused much trouble, and brave Ariomardus who dispensed grief with his arrows, and Seisames the Mysian, and Tharybis, admiral of five times fifty ships, a Lyrnaean by birth and a handsome man, lies wretchedly dead, having enjoyed no very good fortune. And Synnesis, foremost in courage, the leader of the Cilicians, who gave more trouble to the enemy than any other single man, met a glorious end.
All this I report about the commanders; but I have mentioned only a small part of the great suffering that there was.

The list of the Persian dead is apparently modelled on the epic catalogues of slain warriors.[18] However, as it has already been noted, several

[18] E.g. T. Rosenmeyer, *The Art of Aeschylus* (Berkeley: University of California Press, 1982), p. 99ff, 199ff; A.N. Michelini, *Tradition and Dramatic Form in the 'Persians' of Aeschylus* (Leiden: Brill, 1982), p. 15, 99ff; Hall, *Aeschylus. Persians*, pp. 108–109; C.

characteristics of Aeschylus' list contrast with the alleged epic model and instead suggest a comparison with another formal template—the Athenian casualty lists.[19] On the one hand, Aeschylus' list is much more longer than epic catalogues, which usually consist of a few lines only;[20] on the other hand, the 'roll-call of the dead',[21] together with the ethnic,[22] plus in some cases the indication of the military grade and the place of death, clearly resemble the Athenian casualty lists.[23] The use of an epicising language in the description of the Persians' death in battle, which is also usually considered to be a clue to Aeschylus' reference to the epic model,

Dué, *The* Captive *Woman's Lament in Greek Tragedy* (Austin, TX: University of Texas Press, 2006), p. 63.

[19] See M. Ebbott, 'The List of the War Dead in Aeschylus' '*Persians*'', *Harvard Studies in Classical Philology* 100, 2000, 83–96. The date of introduction of the casualty lists in Athens is debated and fluctuates from the Persian wars to the '60s. For a recent and comprehensive treatment of the question, see N.T. Arrington, *Ashes, Images, and Memories: The Presence of the War Dead in Fifth-Century Athens* (Oxford: Oxford University Press, 2015), esp. p. 33ff. In any case, independent from when casualty lists were introduced in Athens, the Athenians surely had familiarity with the type at least since the Marathon battle, as the so-called 'stele of the Marathonomachoi' (*SEG* LVI 430) shows.

[20] E.g. three lines for both the eight men killed by Hector (*Iliad*, V 705ff.) and the nine killed by Patroclus (*Iliad*, XVI 694ff.): epic catalogues of casualties in war feature a high 'onomastic density' (A. Petrovic, 'Casualty Lists in Performance. Name Catalogues and Greek Verse-Inscriptions', in F. Montanari and A. Rengakos (eds), *Dialect, Diction and Style in Greek Literary and Inscribed Epigram* (Berlin-New York: De Gruyter, 2016), pp. 359–88, at 379); according to Petrovic, 'Casualty Lists', 379–81 Aeschylus' catalogue resembles instead another type of Homeric catalogue, e.g. that of the slain warriors enumerated by Nestor to Telemachus (*Od.* III 107–12), which features a lesser onomastic density and offers instead more narrative details. However, the closest example of 'narrativized catalogue' on which Aeschylus' list could have been modelled is that provided by the late Archaic *polyandrion* of Ambrakia (*SEG* XLI 540; see G.F. Randone, 'I distici del *polyandrion* di Ambracia. Un dibattito interrotto', *Acme* 66, 1–2, 2013, 33–52, with previous literature), whose epigram includes a catalogue of war dead's names (ll. 6–10).

[21] M. Anderson, 'The Imagery of the *Persians*', *Greece & Rome* s. II, 19, 1972, 169; Hall, *Aeschylus. Persians,* 132.

[22] The Persians' ethnic basically corresponds to the Athenians' tribal affiliation. See Ebbott, 'List of the War Dead', 89: 'The ethnic identifications of the dead in the Messenger's speech serve a similar function of identifying the political space of these soldiers within the Persian Empire'.

[23] One of the extant Athenian casualty lists preserves all the elements accompanying the name of the dead: tribal affiliation, military grade, and place of battle (*IG* I^3 1162, dated to 449 BC, and referred to the Athenian war dead at the Chersonese, Byzantium, and Hellespontum).

can also be ascribed to Aeschylus' reference to the epigrams for the war dead of Archaic and Classical times, which in turn featured a Homeric lexicon and style.[24] Furthermore, another catalogue, which appears in the *parodos* of the *Persians*, provides a useful internal comparison: at ll. 21–58, when Aeschylus lists the individuals and collectives belonging to the Persian armada, comprising both Persian commanders (ll. 21–32) and allied people (ll. 33–58), he actually provides a catalogue which surely recalls the epic type.[25] The list of Persian war dead in ll. 302–320 instead likely reminded the Athenian audience of their own lists of the war dead.[26] It must also be noted that the emotional effect of the messenger's catalogue may have been even stronger if, as it appears from recent studies, the Athenian casualty lists with the relevant epigrams were commonly read out loud during the public funerary ceremonies for the war dead: as Petrovic observed, 'this play offers evidence of a double performativity: the catalogue of the slain is not only performed on stage to the Athenian audience from the actor's memory, but in the world of

[24] According to D. Korzeniewski, 'Studien zu den *Persen* des Aischylos', part 2, *Helikon* 7, 1967, 27–33, the closing lines of the catalogue (II. 326–28, which provide a graphic vignette of the death of the last mentioned Persian commander, Sinnesis, who εἷς ἀνὴρ πλεῖστον πόνον / ἐχθροῖς παρασχών, εὐκλεῶς ἀπώλετο) closely resemble the typical style of the 'Grabepigram'.

[25] For instance, the catalogues of the ships and the Trojans and their allies in the *Iliad* (II 494–759 and 816–77, respectively). According to Rosenbloom, *Aeschylus: Persians*, 40, the catalogue of the Persian armada 'endows the invasion with epic grandeur'. Garvie, Aeschylus' *Persae*, 161–62, resting on S. Saïd, 'Tragédie et renversement: l'exemple des *Perses*', *Metis* 3, 1988, 321–41, highlights the dramatic relationship, aimed at arousing the audience's sympathy, between the catalogue of the Persian might and the second one listing the dead, where 'each individual death symbolizes the annihilation of the whole contingent' (161). On the contrast between the two catalogues, evoking respectively a massive presence and a palpable absence, see also Rosenbloom, *Aeschylus: Persians*, 40–42, 65–66.

[26] Nonetheless, it must be noted that while the Athenian casualty lists were notoriously aimed at de-individuating the dead and democratically emphasizing the collective, in drama the focus was placed on individuals in order to elicit emotional engagement from the audience. To this purpose, while in the casualty lists, all the information about the fallen's death were given within a common prose-heading or epigram, in Aeschylus' narrativized catalogue, every single individual is introduced together with details about their own military performance, and way and/or place of death.

the play, it is situated in the oral report delivered from the messenger's memory to queen Atossa'.[27]

A further clue suggesting the identification between the Persian dead on the scene and the Athenian fallen comes from the final threnody, where the chorus, in dialogue with Xerxes, cries out the entire city's grief for the loss of its sons (the *kommos* at ll. 931–1077). After Xerxes' evocation of the dead comrades he left behind, the chorus enumerates once again the lost *plethos* (ll. 962–1001):

Ξέρξης ὀλοοὺς ἀπέλειπον Τυρίας ἐκ ναὸς ἔρροντας ἐπ᾿ ἀκταῖς Σαλαμινιάσι, στυφελοῦ θείνοντας ἐπ᾿ ἄκρας.	**Xerxes** I left them dead, Fallen out of a Tyrian ship off the shores, of Salamis, striking against a rugged cape.
Χορός οἰοιοῖ † ποῦ δέ† σοι Φαρνοῦχος κἀριόμαρδός γ᾿ ἀγαθός; ποῦ δὲ Σευάλκης ἄναξ, ἢ Λίλαιος εὐπάτωρ, Μέμφις, Θάρυβις καὶ Μασίστρας, Ἀρτεμβάρης τ᾿ ἠδ᾿ Ὑσταίχμας; τάδε σ᾿ ἐπανερόμαν.	**Chorus** Cry 'oioioi'! Where did you leave Pharnuchus, Yes, and the brave Ariomardus? Where is the lord Seualces, Or the nobly-born Lilaeus, Memphis, Tharybis and Masistras, Artembares and Hystaichmas? I ask you this again!
Ξέρξης ἰὼ, ἰώ μοί τὰς ὠγυγίους κατιδόντες στυγνὰς Ἀθάνας πάντες ἑνὶ πιτύλῳ, ἓ ἕ, ἓ ἕ τλάμονες ἀσπαίρουσι χέρσῳ.	**Xerxes** Ió Ió, ah me! After setting eyes on ancient Athens, Hateful Athens, all of them in one stroke - [*repeated sobs*] gasp their life out wretchedly on the shore!

(continued)

[27] Petrovic, 'Casualty Lists', 381; on the performance of the Athenian casualty lists, see also Ebbott, 'List of the War Dead', 93–94.

(continued)

Χορός ἦ καὶ Περσᾶν τὸν ἄωτον, τὸν σὸν πιστὸν πάντ' ὀφθαλμὸν, μυρία μυρία πεμπαστὰν < ∪ ∪ ∪ ∪ > Βατανώχου, παῖδ' ἄλπιστον τοῦ Σεισάμα τοῦ Μεγαβάτα, Πάρθον τε μέγαν τ' Οἰβάρην ἔλιπες ἔλιπες; ὢ ὢ δαΐων· Πέρσαις ἀγαυοῖς κακὰ πρόκακα λέγεις.	**Chorus** And what of that flower of Persia- Your ever-faithful Eye, Who counted the numberless tens of thousands, < > , the favourite son Of Batanochus The son of Seisames, the son of Megabates, And great Parthus and Oebares- Did you leave them, did you leave them? Oh, oh, hapless ones! You speak of evils beyond evils for noble Persians
Ξέρξης ἴυγγά μοι δῆτ' ἀγαθῶν ἑτάρων ἀνακινεῖς ἄλαστ' ἄλαστα στυγνὰ πρόκακα λέγων βοᾷ βοᾷ μοι μελέων ἔντοσθεν ἦτορ	**Xerxes** You do stir up in me A longing for my brave comrades, Speaking of unforgettable, unforgettable things, hateful Beyond hatefulness My heart cries out, cries out, within my body!
Χορός καὶ μὴν ἄλλους γε ποθοῦμεν, Μάρδων ἀνδρῶν μυριοταγὸν Ξάνθιν, Ἀρίων τ' Ἀγχάρην, Δίαιξίν τ' ἠδ' Ἀρσάκην ἱππιάνακτας, †κηγδαδάταν† καὶ Λυθίμναν Τόλμον τ' αἰχμᾶς ἀκόρεστον. ἔταφον ἔταφον· οὐκ ἀμφὶ σκηναῖς τροχηλάτοισιν ὄπιθεν ἑπομένους.	**Chorus** And there are others too that we miss, Xanthes the commander of ten thousand Mardians Beyond all count; also Arian Anchares, And Anchares of the Arians, And Diaïxis and Arsaces lords of the cavalry, and Egdadates and Lythimnas And Tolmus, never surfeited with battle I am amazed, amazed, that they are not following behind your wheeled tent.

In this second catalogue of the Persian dead, the formal features of the Athenian casualty lists, such as the tribal affiliation and the military grade, are not reproduced; however, we are once again in front of a list of men who died in battle, and survivors (this time not Atossa and the messenger, but Xerxes himself and the chorus of Persian elderly) are mourning. This second list of the Persian fallen, embedded as it is in the chorus' lamentation, provides in my view a further, more explicit clue to understanding the first catalogue as well (*supra*, ll. 303–20). This was not a generic lament for the city,[28] but the collective mourning of the war dead on the stage.[29] The war dead who were mourned were Persian in the scene, but most likely Athenian in the audience's perception.

At a closer glance, the two lamentations of the chorus themselves, mourning the death of their fellow citizens (ll. 256–289 and ll. 908–1077), suggest a possible identification between the audience and the staged situation. Is not the Persian chorus itself indirectly representative of the Athenian civic community, mourning the Athenian war dead all throughout the '70s? Line by line, almost paraphrasing Aeschylus,

[28] The connection of the lament for a fallen city and tragedy has been explored, e.g. in M. Alexiou, *The Ritual Lament in the Greek Tradition* (Cambridge: Cambridge University Press, 1974); H.P. Foley, '*Anodos* Drama: Euripides' *Alcestis* and *Helen*', in R. Hexter and D.L. Selden (eds), *Innovations of Antiquity* (Princeton: Princeton University Press, 1993), pp. 133–60; A. Suter, *Lament: Studies in the Ancient Mediterranean and Beyond* (Oxford: Oxford University Press, 2008), pp. 156–75; M.R. Bachvarova and D.M. Dutsch, 'Mourning a City 'Empty of Men': Stereotypes of Anatolian Communal Lament in Aeschylus' *Persians*', in M.R. Bachvarova, D.M. Dutsch and A. Suter (eds), *The Fall of Cities in the Mediterranean: Commemoration in Literature, Folk-Song and Liturgie* (Cambridge: Cambridge University Press, 2016), pp. 97–105; G. Bakewell, '*Seven Against Thebes*, City Laments, and Athenian History', in Bachvarova, Dutsch and Suter (eds), *The Fall of Cities*, pp. 106–26. However, the lament for the city in tragedy has mostly failed to be interpreted in light of a real context of post-war, inclusive of its peculiar social and emotional dynamics, especially those that can be related to the notion of war trauma. In the case of Aeschylus' *Persians*, the most accredited interpretation (e.g. Hall, *Aeschylus. Persians*, 13; H.P. Foley, *Female Acts in Greek Tragedy* (Princeton: Princeton University Press, 2001), 29), which rests on a conception of the lament as something peculiarly feminine (in any case not irreconcilable with the thesis developed here), holds that the lament of the chorus plays the function of feminizing the Persians, as part of the process of building an antithesis between Greeks and barbarians. *Contra*, Rosenbloom, *Aeschylus: Persians*, 125–26, though with a generally different interpretation, defines the Persian *kommos* as a 'public lament for communal suffering', which fostered the Athenians' identification with the sufferings of the Persians. Similarly, Dué, *The Captive Woman's Lament,* 2006, ch. 2, *passim. Contra* R. Palmisciano, *Dialoghi per voce sola. La cultura del lamento funebre nella Grecia antica* (Roma: Quasar, 2017), 230–32, who denies the possibility of an identification of the Athenians with the Persians who are mourned in the *kommos* of ll. 931–1077.

[29] This interpretation might make sense also in light of the civic calendar, which scheduled the public burial of the war dead during (late?) winter (N. Loraux, *The Invention of Athens. The Funeral Oration in the Classical City* (Cambridge, MA: Harvard University Press, 1986), pp. 37–38), and the tragic performances during the Great Dionysia at the beginning of spring. After the most high expression of public grief on the occasion of the burial of the fallen, tragic catharsis used to provide healing and prepare the civic community to a new beginning.

is not the depiction of the Persian women who have lost their children and husbands in ll. 288–289 suitable to the Athenian women as well? Is not Atossa's eagerness to know Xerxes' fate in ll. 290ss. equal to the anxiety of every Athenian mother, who does not know whether she will ever embrace her son again?[30] How many Athenians would have been slammed against the cliffs as the Persian Artembares? How many Athenians would have fallen from the ships as Dadaces, or Arcteus, Adeues and Pheresseues? How many Athenian corpses would have been pushed back by the waves to the Salamis coasts, as Lilaeus, Arsames, and Argestes? How many Athenians would have found themselves with a blood-drenched beard as Matallus of Chrysa? Also, in the chorus' lament in ll. 537–40, do not the Persian women (who are said to be *pollai*, not to exclude any role in the family ties), tearing their veils apart and imbuing their vests with tears, impersonate every Athenian mother, sister, and wife who have lost their men? And does not the closer focus on the young Persian women mourning their newly wed husbands in ll. 541–45 work as a touching insight into the intimate desperation of every young Athenian widow?

Last but not least, does not Xerxes himself, with his clothes torn off and his desperation for having lost his compatriots in battle, as it is depicted in the final section of the play, embody every Athenian veteran, who had come back home pained and possibly even shocked, and was now sitting in the theatre attending the *Persians*? In other terms, does not Xerxes' *nostos* represent every Athenian veteran's homecoming? In addition to this, Xerxes' dramatic cry at the very end of the play seems to explicate the very key for understanding the ultimate meaning of this whole representation (ll. 1074–77):[31]

[30] On the centrality of Atossa in framing Xerxes' return from war and defining the relationship mother-son in terms of loss, see L. McClure, 'Maternal Authority and Heroic Disgrace in Aeschylus's *Persae*', *Transactions of the American Philological Association* 136, 2006, 71–97.

[31] I would consider the possibility that part of a destroyed trireme, or a symbolic object representative of a trireme, was physically present on the stage in the final part of the play. On the importance of 'objects as actors' on the Athenian stage, see M. Müller, *Objects as Actors: Props and the Poetics of Performance in Greek Tragedy* (Chicago: University of Chicago Press, 2016).

Ξέρξης	**Xerxes**
ἠὴ ἠὴ τρισκάλμοισιν-	Ehhh-ehhh, ehhh-ehhh-the triple-oared
Χορός	**Chorus**
ἠὴ ἠή, βάρισιν ὀλόμενοι.	Ehhh-ehhh, ehhh-ehhh-boats destroyed them!
Ξέρξης	**Xerxes**
< >	< Escort me now to my palace.>
Χορός	**Chorus**
πέμψω τοί σε δυσθρόοις γόοις.	Yes, I will escort you, with loud wails of grief.

Here the symbols *par excellence* of the Greek victory at Salamis, the Athenian triremes, are depicted as funeral wagons. The scene is powerful, and rich in tragic irony. On the one hand, the visualization of the protagonists of the Greek triumph over the Persians would have stirred the Athenian national pride; on the other hand, the depiction of the triremes as funeral carts carrying war dead must have brought to completion the audience's empathy: in light of the, here, developed analysis of the tragedy, we might in fact assume that people sitting in the theatre likely perceived the Persian dead carried onto the triremes as their own dead. Fortunately, they were not.

Collective War Trauma and Tragic Catharsis

Aeschylus' thematic choice, the sufferings of the Persians for the copious casualties at Salamis, perfectly fits the tragic mechanism of the catharsis, which envisaged first the acknowledgement of the analogy between ones' own personal condition and that on the stage, and secondly the awareness that it might have been them on the stage, but they are not: the evocation of their own casualty lists through the two Persians' catalogues, as well as the description of the pains suffered by both who fell in war and who survived, led the Athenians to recognize the analogy with their present tragedy of war casualties, allowing them to reach therapeutic detachment.

I suggest therefore that the play does not only contain the lamentation for the city following a massive fatality, as it has already been—and in any case rightly—argued.[32] It works in fact as a therapy against what

[32] The two plays are paired and analysed both in their reciprocal connection and in their relationship with an alleged near Eastern archetype in Bachvrarova-Dutsch, *The Fall of Cities*. Their study, although with different aims, also focuses on the function of the two plays (especially their respective choruses) as representative of the genre of public

can be labelled as a *collective war trauma*, which involves the whole civic community and is connected to the substantial war casualties and related sufferings they had experienced and still have to cope with. The analysis of Aeschylus' *Persians* as it has been developed above lies somewhat in the middle between the two current approaches to war trauma, the psychological and the historical one: on the one hand, it deals with an important aspect related to the individual phenomenology of war trauma as it is experienced today in the theatrical projects for veterans, i.e. tragedy as a therapeutic means of catharsis,[33] ultimately resting on Aristotle's theory of tragic catharsis;[34] on the other hand, it refers to a collective trauma in its widely cultural and historical dimension.[35]

Aeschylus' play effectively worked as a form of cultural therapy against war trauma in post-war Athens. After the initial identification, provoked by the acknowledgement of an analogy between the audience and the stage, and a sympathetic identification, a 'filter' (if the tragedian had chosen a right one) induced the detachment, which was required in order to reach the catharsis. However, the cathartic process did not involve the single individuals, whose psychological conditions are admittedly irrecoverable for us, but the whole civic community. Subject to the methodological recommendations given above, war trauma does appear

lamentation for a major military catastrophe, therefore as a collective response on account of massive fatalities. Garvie, *Aeschylus'* Persae, xi: 'Phrynichus' *Capture of Miletus* was so upsetting because the tragic suffering was too direct and too close to home. The two Salamis plays [both Phrynichus' *Phoenissae* and Aeschylus' *Persians*] were more successful no doubt partly because the Athenians were the victors in the battle. And yet, as we shall see, they were still able to identify with the losers in their suffering.

[33] See *supra*, n.4.

[34] Nonetheless, it must be noted that, among the extensive bibliography concerning the cathartic function of ancient tragedy, M. Berzins McCoy, *Wounded Heroes: Vulnerability as a Virtue in Ancient Greek Literature and Philosophy* (Oxford: Oxford University Press, 2013), esp. ch. 7, offers an interpretation of Aristotle's notion of tragic catharsis as a form of rebalancing not only of an individual soul, but of the community at large, with useful hints for the analysis of the function of drama as a form of cultural therapy. This reading fits with the here proposed interpretation of Aeschylus' *Persians*.

[35] Admittedly, since we possess no critical or anecdotal responses to tragedy from the fifth century (except for Phrynichus' *Sack of Miletus*: see *supra*, n. 15), it is exactly from the treatment of individual war trauma through ancient tragedy today that we can assume that 'Athenian tragedy offered a form of performance-based collective 'catharsis' or 'cultural therapy' by providing a place where the traumatic experiences faced by the spectators were reflected upon the gaze of the masked characters performing before them' (Meineck, 'Combat Trauma', 7).

as a fertile field of investigation where to test an interdisciplinary and comparative dialogue between the ancient and the contemporary world.

Acknowledgements I want to thank Jason Crowley and Owen Rees for their wonderful hospitality in Manchester, and the organization of a great workshop with stimulating discussions in a friendly atmosphere. I am also grateful for their valuable comments on this essay, and the commitment of the editors to the publication of this volume. Last but not least, I would like to thank Bernd Steinbock for sharing his expertise on social memory and trauma with me and commenting on the draft of this paper with important suggestions.

Bibliography

Alexander, J.C. et al., *Cultural Trauma and Collective Identity* (Berkeley: University of California Press, 2004).

Alexander, J.C., *Trauma. A Social Theory* (Cambridge: Cambridge University Press, 2012).

Alexiou, M., *The Ritual Lament in the Greek Tradition* (Cambridge: Cambridge University Press, 1974).

Allan, W. and Kelly, A., 'Listening to Many Voices: Greek Tragedy as Popular Art', in A. Marmodoro and J. Hill (eds), *The Author's Voice in Classical and Late Antiquity* (Oxford: Oxford University Press, 2013), pp. 77–122.

Anderson, M., 'The Imagery of the *Persians*', *Greece & Rome* s. II, 19, 1972, 166–74.

Arrington, N. T., *Ashes, Images, and Memories: The Presence of the War Dead in Fifth-Century Athens* (Oxford: Oxford University Press, 2015).

Bachvarova, M.R. and D.M. Dutsch, 'Mourning a City 'Empty of Men': Stereotypes of Anatolian Communal Lament in Aeschylus' *Persians*', in M.R. Bachvarova, D.M. Dutsch and A. Suter (eds), *The Fall of Cities in the Mediterranean: Commemoration in Literature, Folk-Song and Liturgie* (Cambridge: Cambridge University Press, 2016), pp. 97–105.

Bakewell, G., '*Seven Against Thebes*, City Laments, and Athenian History', in M.R. Bachvarova, D.M. Dutsch and A. Suter (eds), *The Fall of Cities in the Mediterranean: Commemoration in Literature, Folk-Song and Liturgie* (Cambridge: Cambridge University Press, 2016), pp. 106–26.

Bearzot, C., 'Le conseguenze della guerra nell'antichità', *Studium* 111, 2015, 95–106.

Berzins McCoy, M., *Wounded Heroes: Vulnerability as a Virtue in Ancient Greek Literature and Philosophy* (Oxford: Oxford University Press, 2013).

Brunner J. and Zajde, N. *Holocaust und Trauma: kritische Perspektiven zur Entstehung und Wirkung eines Paradigmas* (Göttingen: Wallstein, 2011).

Cathy, C. (ed), *Trauma: Explorations in Memory* (Baltimore: John Hopkins University Press, 1995).

Cathy, C., *Unclaimed Experience: Trauma, Narrative and History* (Baltimore: John Hopkins University Press, 216).

Caston V. and S.-M. Weineck, (eds), *Our Ancient Wars: Rethinking War through the Classics* (Ann Arbor: University of Michigan Press, 2016).

Cosmopoulos, M., (ed), *Experiencing War. Trauma and Society from Ancient Greece to the Iraq War* (Chicago Ill: Ares, 2007).

Crowley, J., *The Psychology of the Athenian Hoplite. The Culture of Combat in Classical Athens* (Cambridge: Cambridge University Press, 2012).

Crowley, J., 'Beyond the Universal Soldier: Combat Trauma in Classical Antiquity', in P. Meineck and D. Konstan (eds), *Combat Trauma and the Ancient Greeks* (New York: Palgrave, 2014), pp. 105–30.

Crocq, M.A. and Crocq, L., 'From Shell Shock and War Neurosis to Post-traumatic Stress Disorder: A History of Psychotraumatology', *Dialogues in Clinical Neurosciences* 2.1, 2000, 47–55.

Doerries, B., *Theatre of War: What Ancient Greek Tragedies Can Teach Us Today* (New York: Scribe, 2015).

Dué, C., *The Captive Woman's Lament in Greek Tragedy* (Austin, TX: University of Texas Press, 2006).

Easterling, P.E., 'Anachronism in Greek Tragedy', *Journal of Hellenistic Studies*1985, 105, 1–10.

Easterling, P.E., 'Constructing the Heroic', in C.B.R. Pelling (ed), *Greek Tragedy and the Historian* (Oxford: Clarendon Press, 1997), pp. 21–37.

Ebbott, M., 'The List of the War Dead in Aeschylus' "*Persians*"', *Harvard Studies in Classical Philology* 100, 2000, 83–96.

Foley, H.P., 'Anodos Drama: Euripides' *Alcestis* and *Helen*', in R. Hexter and D.L. Selden (eds), *Innovations of Antiquity* (Princeton: Princeton University Press, 1993), pp. 133–60.

Foley, H.P., *Female Acts in Greek Tragedy* (Princeton: Princeton University Press, 2001).

Gabriel, R.A., *The Madness of Alexander the Great and the Myth of the Military Genius* (Barnsley: Pen & Sword, 2015).

Garland, R., *Athens Burning. The Persian Invasion of Greece and the Evacuation of Attica* (Baltimore: John Hopkins University Press, 2016).

Garvie, A.F. (ed), *Aeschylus'* Persae, *with Introduction and Commentary* (Oxford: Oxford University Press, 2009).

Hall, E., *Inventing the Barbarian: Greek Self-Definition Through Tragedy* (Oxford: Clarendon Press, 1989).

Hall, E., (ed), *Aeschylus. Persians* (Warminster: Aris and Phillips, 1996).

Harrison, T., *The Emptiness of Asia. Aeschylus'* Persians *and the History of the Fifth Century* (London: Bloomsbury, 2000).

Hirsch, M. and Spitzer, L., 'The Witness in the Archive: Holocaust Studies/Memory Studies', in S. Radstone and B. Schwarz (eds), *Memory. Histories, Theories, Debates* (New York: Fordham University Press, 2010), pp. 390–405.

Hirschberger, G., 'Collective Trauma and the Social Construction of Meaning', *Frontiers in Psychology* 9, 2018, 1–18.

Hopman, M., 'Layered Stories in Aeschylus' *Persians*', in J. Grethlein and A. Rengakos (eds), *Narratology and Interpretation: The Content of Narrative Form in Ancient Literature* (Berlin and New York: Walter de Gruyter, 2009), pp. 357–76.

Hunt, N. (2010), *Memory, War and Trauma* (Cambridge: Cambridge University Press, 2010).

Hunt, P., 'Athenian Militarism and Recourse to War', in D. Pritchard (ed), *War, Democracy and Culture in Classical Athens* (Cambridge: Cambridge University Press, 2010), pp. 225–42.

Kellermann, N., 'Transmitted Holocaust Trauma: Curse or Legacy? The Aggravating and Mitigating Factors of Holocaust Transmission', *The Israel Journal of Psychiatry and Related Science* 45, 2008, 263–71.

King, H., 'Recovering Hysteria from History: Herodotus and the First Case of 'Shell-Shock'', in P. Halligan, C. Bass and J.C. Marshall (eds), *Contemporary Approaches to the Science of Hysteria: Clinical and Theoretical Perspectives* (Oxford: Oxford University Press, 2001), pp. 36–48.

Korzeniewski, D., 'Studien zu den *Persern* des Aischylos', part 2, *Helikon* 7, 1967, 27–62.

La Capra, D., *Writing History, Writing Trauma* (Baltimore and London: John Hopkins University Press, 2001).

Leys, R., *Trauma. A Genealogy* (Chicago: Chicago University Press, 2000).

Lockwood, T., 'The Political Theorizing of Aeschylus' *Persians*', *Interpretations* 43, 2017, 383–401.

Loraux, N., *The Invention of Athens. The Funeral Oration in the Classical City* (Cambridge, MA: Harvard University Press, 1986).

Luckhurst, R., *The Trauma Question* (London: Routledge, 2008).

McClure, L., 'Maternal Authority and Heroic Disgrace in Aeschylus's *Persae*', *Transactions of the American Philological Association* 136, 2006, 71–97.

Meineck, P., 'Combat Trauma and the Tragic Stage: 'Restoration' by Cultural Catharsis', *Intertexts* 16.1, 2012, 7–24.

Meineck, P., 'Thebes as High-Collateral-Damage Target. Moral Accountability for Killing in Aeschylus' *Seven against Thebes*', in I. Torrance (ed), *Aeschylus and War: Comparative Perspectives on* Seven Against Thebes (Abingdon, Oxon: Rouledge, 2017), pp. 49–70.

Meineck, P. and D. Konstan (eds), *Combat Trauma and the Ancient Greeks* (New York, 2014).

Michelini, A.N., *Tradition and Dramatic Form in the 'Persians' of Aeschylus* (Leiden: Brill, 1982).

Mills, S., 'Ektos Sumphoras: Tragic Athens', *Polis* 34, 2017, 208–25.

Mills, S., *Drama, Oratory and Thucydides in Fifth-Century Athens: Teaching Imperial Lessons* (London: Routldege, 2020).

Müller, M., *Objects as Actors: Props and the Poetics of Performance in Greek Tragedy* (Chicago: University of Chicago Press, 2016).

Palaima, T.G., 'Courage and Prowess Afoot in Homer and the Vietnam of Tim O'Brien', *Classical and Modern Literature* 20.3, 2000, 1–22.

Palaima, T.G., 'When War Is Performed, What Do Soldiers and Veterans Want to Hear and See and Why', in P. Meineck and D. Konstan (eds), *Combat Trauma and the Ancient Greeks* (New York: Palgrave, 2014), pp. 261–85.

Palaima, T.G., 'War Stories Told, Untold and Retold from Troy to Tinian to Fort Campbell,' *Arion* 23.3, 2016, 1–33.

Palmisciano, R., *Dialoghi per voce sola. La cultura del lamento funebre nella Grecia antica* (Roma: Quasar, 2017).

Payen, P., *Les revers de la guerre en Grèce ancienne: histoire et historiographie* (Paris: Belin, 2012).

Pelling, C., 'Aeschylus' *Persae* and History', in C. Pelling (ed), *Greek Tragedy and the Historian* (Oxford: Clarendon Press, 1997), pp. 1–19.

Petrovic A., 'Casualty Lists in Performance. Name Catalogues and Greek Verse-Inscriptions', in F. Montanari and A. Rengakos (eds), *Dialect, Diction and Style in Greek Literary and Inscribed Epigram* (Berlin-New York: De Gruyter, 2016), pp. 359–88.

Pritchard, D.M., 'The Symbiosis between Democracy and War: The Case of Ancient Athens', in D.M. Pritchard (ed), *War, Democracy and Culture in Classical Athens* (Cambridge: Cambridge University Press, 2010), pp. 1–62.

Proietti, G., 'Fare i conti con la guerra. Forme del discorso civico ad Atene nel V secolo', in E. Franchi and G. Proietti (eds), *Conflict in Communities. Forward-looking Memories in Classical Athens* (Trento: Trento University Press, 2017), pp. 69–108.

Proietti, G., 'Can an Ancient Truth Become an Old Lie? A Few Methodological Remarks Concerning Current Comparative Research on War and Its Aftermath', in M. Giangiulio, E. Franchi and G. Proietti (eds), *Commemorating War and War Dead. Ancient and Modern* (Stuttgart: Franz Steiner Verlag, 2019), pp. 71–92.

Proietti, G., 'Athens as a 'Landscape of Trauma': Phrynichus' *Sack of Miletus* and the Aftermath of the Persian Wars', in L. Cecchet, Ch. Degelmann and M. Patzelt (eds), *Impact of War on the Home Front in the Ancient World* (Cambridge: Cambridge University Press, 2019), pp. 79–98.

Raaflaub, K.A., 'War and the City: The Brutality of War and its Impact on the Community', in P. Meineck and D. Konstan (eds), *Combat Trauma and the Ancient Greeks* (New York: Palgrave, 2014), pp. 15–46.

Raaflaub, K.A., '*Lysistrata* and War's Impact on the Home Front', in V. Caston and S.-M. Weineck (eds), *Our Ancient Wars. Rethinking War through the Classics* (Ann Arbor: University of Michigan Press, 2016), pp. 38–74.

Randone, G.F., 'I distici del *polyandrion* di Ambracia. Un dibattito interrotto', *Acme* 66.1–2, 2013, 33–52.

Rees, O., 'We Need to Talk about Epizelus: 'PTSD' and the Ancient World', *Medical Humanities* 46.1, 2019, 46–54.

Rees, O., *Military Departures, Homecomings and Death in Classical Athens. Hoplite Transitions* (London: Bloomsbury, 2022).

Retief, P., 'The Army of Alexander the Great and Combat Stress Syndrome (326 BC)', *Acta Theologica* 7, 2005, 29–43.

Roisman, H.M., (ed), *The Encyclopedia of Greek Tragedy* (Oxford: Oxford University Press, 2014).

Roisman, J., 'On Phrynichos' *Sack of Miletus* and *Phoinissai*', *Eranos* 86, 1988, 15–23.

Rosenbloom, D. (ed), *Aeschylus: Persians* (London: Duckworth, 2006).

Rosenmeyer, T., *The Art of Aeschylus* (Berkeley: University of California Press, 1982).

Saïd, S., 'Tragédie et renversement: l'exemple des *Perses*', *Metis* 3, 1988, 321–41.

Shay, J., *Achilles in Vietnam: Combat Trauma and the Undoing of Character* (New York: Atheneum, 1995).

Shay, J., *Odysseus in America. Combat Trauma and the Trials of Homecoming* (New York: Scribner, 2002).

Shay, J., 'Homer's Leaders in America's Forces: Leadership and Prevention of Psychological and Moral Injury', in M. Cosmopoulos (ed), *Experiencing War. Trauma and Society from Ancient Greece to the Iraq War* (Chicago: Ares, 2007), pp. 258–77.

Shephard, B., *A War of Nerves. Soldiers and Psychiatrists in the Twentieth Century* (Cambridge, MA: Harvard University Press, 2001).

Sommerstein, Alan H. (ed and trans), *Persians. Seven Against Thebes. Supplicants. Prometheus* (Cambridge, MA: Harvard University Press, 2008).

Sourvinou-Inwood C., *Tragedy and Athenian Religion* (Lanham MD.: Lexington Books, 2003).

Steinbock, B., 'Sufferings Too Great for Tears. The Destruction of the Athenian Expeditionary Corps in Sicily', in M. Jonasch (ed), *The Fight for Greek Sicily. Society, Politics, and Landscape* (Oxford: Oxbow Books, 2020), pp. 73–98.

Suter, A., *Lament: Studies in the Ancient Mediterranean and Beyond* (Oxford: Oxford University Press, 2008).

Tritle, L.A., *From Melos to My Lai. War and Survival* (London: Routledge, 2000).
Tritle, L.A., 'Alexander and the Killing of Cleitus the Black', in W. Heckel and L.A. Tritle (eds), *Crossroads of History: The Age of Alexander* (Claremont: Regina Books, 2003), pp. 127–46.
Tritle, L.A., 'Xenophon's Portrait of Clearchus. A Study in Post-Traumatic Stress Disorder', in C. Tuplin (ed), *Xenophon and his World* (Stuttgart: Franz Steiner Verlag, 2004), pp. 325–39.
Tritle, L.A., 'Gorgias, the Encomium of Helen, and the Trauma of War', *Clio's Psyche* 16.2, 2009, 195–99.
Tritle, L.A., "Ravished Minds' in the Ancient World', in P. Meineck and D. Konstan (eds), *Combat Trauma and the Ancient Greeks* (New York: Palgrave, 2014), pp. 87–103.

Combat Trauma and Ajax: A Script-Based Approach

Constantine Christoforou

This chapter engages with the ongoing debate between the 'Universalists'[1] and the 'Relativists'[2] regarding the experience of combat trauma in the ancient world by positing a new, culturally determined form of combat trauma using Sophocles' *Ajax* as a case study. By 'trauma', I am referring

[1] By 'Universalists', I refer to scholars who take the experience of combat trauma to be universal. See J. Shay, *Achilles in Vietnam, Combat Trauma and the Undoing of Character* (New York: Pocket Books, 1994);

J. Shay, *Odysseus in America. Combat Trauma and the Trials of Homecoming* (New York: Scribner, 2003); L.A. Tritle, *From Melos to My Lai, War and Survival* (London: Routledge, 2000); and L.A. Tritle, '"Ravished Minds" in the Ancient World', in P. Meineck and D. Konstan (eds), *Combat Trauma and the Ancient Greeks*. (London: Palgrave, 2014), pp. 87–104 for examples of scholars who apply this to ancient Greek warfare.

[2] By 'Relativists', I refer to scholars who take the experience of trauma to be heavily influenced by society and culture, meaning the experience of trauma is not universal. See specifically the work of Jason Crowley: J. Crowley, *The Psychology of the Athenian Hoplite: The culture of Combat in Classical Athens* (Cambridge: Cambridge University Press, 2012), and J. Crowley, 'Beyond the Universal Soldier: Combat Trauma in Classical Antiquity', in P. Meineck and D. Konstan (eds), *Combat Trauma and the Ancient Greeks*. (London: Palgrave, 2014), pp. 105–130.

C. Christoforou (✉)
University of Roehampton, London, UK
e-mail: christoc1@roehampton.ac.uk

O. Rees et al. (eds.), *Combat Stress in Pre-modern Europe*, Mental Health in Historical Perspective,
https://doi.org/10.1007/978-3-031-09947-2_4

to an extremely distressing experience, which in this case is driven by a loss of military honour. In this sense, I refer to the experience as 'combat trauma'. I am not equating Ajax's experience to any modern medical or psychological experience of Post-Traumatic Stress Disorder (PTSD), or any similar diagnosis.

Recent developments in the field of Emotion Studies have demonstrated that analysing 'Scripts' provides the most well-rounded account of a given culture's emotional experiences. A script-based methodology aims to create a narrative by piecing together the sequence of emotional responses and reactions by the individual within their cultural context. By utilising a script-based methodology, I argue that while Ajax's emotional experience is often attributed to PTSD, he is in fact displaying an ancient Greek script triggered by a loss of honour. Ajax feels dishonoured as he is not awarded the arms of Achilles which he feels that he has the right to. Traumatised by this, Ajax is overcome with rage.[3] Ajax then commits torturous acts on (what he believes to be) the Greek generals; after this, Ajax's rage cools and he contemplates a life without honour.[4] Realising that such a life has no meaning, Ajax falls on his sword in an attempt to restore a part of his lost honour, and to get his final revenge on the Greeks.[5]

I begin this chapter by critiquing both the 'Universalist' and 'Relativist' approaches to the myth. I then separate Ajax's tragic madness from the script I am presenting—which is a trauma driven by a loss of honour. Following this, I provide an explanation of the script-based methodology and how it can help enhance our reading of Ajax's emotional experience. After this, I analyse the script of Ajax. I first scrutinise Ajax's emotional response to losing out on the arms, followed by a consideration of his violent act of revenge, I then offer a reading of his subsequent shame and contemplation of a life without honour, and finish by analysing the significance of his suicide.

As this play concerns a warrior who suffers from 'madness' and eventually takes his own life, it has drawn the attention of scholars, ex-soldiers, and playwrights who wish to make comparisons between the ancient and

[3] Sophocles, *Ajax*, 41.

[4] Sophocles, *Ajax* 55, 479–80.

[5] Sophocles, *Ajax*, 865.

modern experience of PTSD.[6] However, both a Universalist and a Relativist interpretation of Ajax's experience fail to provide a full picture of the emotional experience of Ajax. Lawrence Tritle, who adopts a Universalist position claimed that Ajax was 'driven to suicide as a result of battle induced trauma'.[7] Tritle argues that Ajax's rage, violent outburst, and consequent suicide was driven by the loss of his friend Achilles, rather than Ajax losing the judgement of the arms of Achilles. Crucially, Tritle concludes that this interpretation would offer a plausible explanation for Ajax's behaviour.[8] The issue here is that Tritle is searching for a plausible explanation for a twentieth-century American audience; this would not be a plausible explanation to the ancient Greeks. As a Universalist however, Tritle is not required to pay attention to fifth-century Greek thought and custom. To Universalists, PTSD is a universal phenomenon meaning that an individual is affected regardless of society or culture. A fifth-century Athenian would be affected just as a twentieth-century American would—the experience is universal. Using this approach, we fail to appreciate the complexity of PTSD and ignore the different manifestations, experiences, and articulations of both events, and their emotional impact on individuals that can derive from differing cultures.

The limitations of Universalism are addressed by Jason Crowley, who adopts a Relativist position. Crowley argues that to diagnose an ancient Greek with PTSD would be to 'ignore the vast social, religious, and tactical differences that separate the modern from the ancient world'.[9] However, I would argue that though Ajax may not have been suffering from PTSD per se, he is suffering from a culturally determined form of trauma. Specifically, Crowley argues that battlefield bravery 'both defined a man and determined his social worth'.[10] He uses this observation to

[6] See for example Tritle, *From Melos to My Lai*; T. Wertenbaker, *Our Ajax* (London: Faber & Faber, 2013); B. Doerries, *The Theater of War: What Ancient Greek Tragedies Can Teach Us Today*. (New York: Knopf, 2015). For a discussion of modern productions of Ajax and PTSD see E. Cole, 'Post-Traumatic Stress Disorder and the Performance Reception of Sophocles' *Ajax*', in D. Stuttard (ed), *Looking at Ajax* (London: Bloomsbury, 2019), pp. 151–60.

[7] Tritle, *From Melos to My Lai*, p. 75.

[8] Ibid., p. 188.

[9] J. Crowley, and O. Rees, 'PTSD in Ancient Greece: Was There Mental Trauma in Ancient Warfare?' in J. Brouwers (ed), *Ancient Warfare IX.4* (Rotterdam: Karwansaray Publishers, 2013), p. 74.

[10] Crowley, 'Beyond the Universal Soldier', p. 111.

suggest that the Greeks embraced killing, death, and battle as it led to them being rewarded with honour and glory. However, Ajax is a man who is recognised as second only to Achilles for his bravery on the battlefield but is *denied* the recognition, honour, and glory that he deserves. This lack of recognition would be traumatic to Ajax. If Ajax fights his whole life for honour and glory but his achievements are unacknowledged, then socially his life has no meaning. He must then go to great lengths in order to restore his honour and this leads to his extreme act of violent revenge. In order to understand Ajax's experience, we should try to understand the depiction of Ajax in terms of fifth-century Greek thought and custom, understanding how and why something may be traumatic to an ancient Greek rather than attempting to find similarities with modern patient's experience of PTSD.

To fully understand Ajax's emotional experience, it is crucial to separate his tragic madness (which is a delusion sent from Athena 51–52) from his rage and murderous intent.[11] I argue against the theory that Ajax is 'mad' throughout the play.[12] There are two storylines running parallel in this play: one is a classic tragic storyline, Ajax refuses the help of Athena at Troy, Athena inflicts Ajax with madness as punishment, the power of the Gods is demonstrated. Running parallel to this storyline is the script of Ajax's emotional experience following his loss of honour: Ajax is angry because he has lost his honour, he plans a murderous revenge, fails, and takes his own life in an attempt to restore his honour. Reginald Winnington-Ingram argues that Ajax's madness was 'something which has

[11] For tragic madness, see A. Obrien-Moore, *Madness in Ancient Literature* (Weimar: R. Wahner Sohn, 1924).

B. Simon, *Mind and Madness in Ancient Greece: The Classical Roots in Modern Psychiatry* (Ithaca: Cornell University Press, 1978); R. Padel, *In and Out of the Mind: Greek Images of the Tragic Self* (Princeton: Princeton University Press, 1994); R. Padel, *Whom Gods Destroy: Elements of Greek and Tragic Madness* (Princeton: Princeton University Press, 1995); A. Thiher, *Revels in Madness: Insanity in Medicine and Literature* (Ann Arbor: University of Michigan Press, 1999); C. Thumiger, *Hidden Paths, Self and Characterisation in Greek Tragedy: Euripides Bacchae* (London: Institute of Classical Studies, 2007); B. Holmes, *The Symptom and the Subject: The Emergence of the Physical Body in Ancient Greece* (Princeton: Princeton University Press, 2010); J. Pegler, *Curing Madness* (London: Chipmunka Publishing, 2011); V.W. Harris (ed), *Mental Disorders in the Classical World* (Leiden: Brill, 2013).

[12] R.P. Winnington-Ingram, *Sophocles: An Interpretation* (Cambridge: Cambridge University Press, 1980).

grown with Ajax during his life span, something that his life has bred'.[13] He labels Ajax a megalomaniac and states that 'the seeds of madness were already in him'.[14] However, this does not fit with fifth-century Athenian ideas regarding madness. As Ruth Padel argues, the ancient Greeks had no concept of long-term madness; being mad required physical symptoms, once those symptoms had disappeared, you were deemed sane.[15] Therefore, the concept of Ajax being mad throughout the play would not have been fathomable.

Ajax's 'madness' came from Athena. No one in the audience would have questioned this due to the fact that Athena alters Ajax's vision—a typical symptom of tragic madness. The Greeks did not separate visual perception from thinking, and within the play, Sophocles uses the verbs meaning 'see' as synonyms for 'know'. For example, Odysseus says that he now sees (ὁρῶ) that mortals are nothing but phantoms meaning that he *knows* because he *sees*.[16] Therefore, by Athena affecting Ajax's ability to see, she affects his mental state. Athena turns Ajax insane, and once Ajax can see things for what they are again he is sane; he is not 'mad' throughout. This is why his desire to murder the Greeks must be separated from his altered vision during his bout of tragic madness sent from Athena. His murderous intent due to his lost honour is with him before Athena intervenes, and remains with him until his death: it is consistent, unlike his temporary bout of tragic madness which leaves him once Athena reinstates his vision. In summation, his desire to murder the generals would not have been viewed as 'mad' by a fifth-century audience. Ajax's dishonour has caused a rage to grow inside him, and this is distinguishable from his madness which is sent by Athena. When viewed in relation to ancient Greek notions of madness, he is insane when under the spell of Athena, and once this is lifted, he is sane once again.

As I have demonstrated, clarity is needed when deciphering the emotional experience of Ajax. In order to provide this clarity, I utilise a script-based approach. For my understanding of scripts and their relationship to ancient Greek culture, I have considered the observations and

[13] Ibid., p. 38.

[14] Ibid, p. 41.

[15] See Padel, *Whom Gods Destroy*, chapter 4, regarding temporary vs long term madness.

[16] See M. Simpson, 'Sophocles' Ajax: His Madness and Transformation', *Arethusa* 2.1, 1969, 88–103. For specific examples of Sophocles using 'see' as know', see n. 9.

explanations offered by Sanders, Cairns, and Kaster.[17] Scripts are narratives of emotional scenarios; they will as Cairns explains 'encompass (at least) the conditions in which emotion X occurs, the perceptions and appraisals of those conditions, and the responses (whether symptomatic, expressive, or pragmatic) that result'.[18] This allows us to analyse an ancient source 'without subjecting it to the distortions either of unreflective modern assumptions or of revisionary scientific theory'.[19] Looking at the ancient source first and creating a narrative of particular emotional scenarios that appear, rather than attempting to find our own preconceived ideas of emotions within ancient Greek sources, allows us to uncover a more accurate depiction of ancient emotion.

As Sanders notes, there are certain primary emotions which can be regarded as transhistorical: such as anger, however, what *causes* anger can differ greatly from culture to culture. He stresses that secondary emotions (envy and jealousy for his particular study) 'are thought to be more socially complex and therefore develop later as a child learns the social rules of their culture'.[20] Honour and shame, much like envy and jealousy, would be heavily influenced by the social context to which they belong. Therefore, in order to analyse the emotional response of Ajax, it is essential to read his experience as a narrative within the parameters of fifth-century Athenian ideas regarding honour and shame. An attempt to read the play using modern psychological approaches to combat trauma or modern ideas regarding anger, revenge, honour, and shame would be inadequate. Studying the script of Ajax's emotional experience through the consideration of ancient Greek concepts such as *hybris*,[21] *time*,[22] and *aidos*[23] provides a more well-rounded explanation. Ajax loses the award

[17] R.A. Kaster, *Emotion, Restraint and Community in Ancient Rome* (Oxford: Oxford University Press, 2005); D. Cairns, 'Look both ways: Studying Emotion in Ancient Greece', *Critical Quarterly* 50.4, 2008, 43–62; E. Sanders, *Envy and Jealousy in Classical Greece: A Socio-Psychological Approach* (Oxford: Oxford University Press, 2014).

[18] Cairns, 'Look Both Ways', 46.

[19] Ibid., 46.

[20] Sanders, *Envy and Jealousy*, p. 3.

[21] I take *hybris* to mean a mortal who oversteps the mark due to excessive pride and does not understand his status and limitations. More is said on the concept below.

[22] I translate *time* as the concept of honour, or an appreciation of one's worth.

[23] The concept of shame, D. Cairns, *Aidos, the Psychology and Ethics of Honour and Shame in Ancient Greek Literature* (Oxford: Clarendon Press, 1993).

of Achilles' arms and views this as an act of *hybris* against him. This leads to him feeling *atimia* and stirred up within him a desire for revenge. This revenge leads to him planning and committing an act of *hybris* of his own in an attempt to regain his lost honour. His attempt is futile, and he resorts to death by suicide after being overwhelmed by *aidos* and a desire for revenge. Studying this narrative closely, paying attention to concepts such as *hybris*, *time*, and *aidos*, brings us closer to a view of Ajax's emotional experience within its historical context.

Although modern scholars interpret the play as follows[24]:Ajax served at war, Ajax 'went mad', Ajax dies by suicide—this is a misinterpretation of the text. By analysing Ajax's experience with regard to fifth-century thought and custom, we get closer to uncovering how Ajax suffered and how this suffering was articulated. Instead, I identify the following script: Ajax is dishonoured after not being awarded the arms of Achilles which has traumatised him, he was then overcome with rage and committed torturous acts on what he thought to be the Greek generals, he decided to take his own life in order to restore as much of his lost honour as possible and to enact revenge on the Greek commanders.

The first stage of Ajax's emotional experience is described by Athena as she explains Ajax is: 'Oppressed by anger because of the arms of Achilles'.[25] Ajax is experiencing a strong form of anger due to losing the judgement of the arms. He is particularly angry because he feels the Greeks have dishonoured him by denying him the arms, he gives as an explanation for killing them: 'So that never again shall they **refuse honour** to Ajax'.[26] This dishonour stems from the fact that Ajax thinks that the Greeks are denying him something which he has the rights to: 'If Achilles were alive and had been going to award the victory for supreme valour in a contest for his own arms, no one else would have seized them instead of me'.[27]

Within its ancient Athenian dramatic context, Ajax would have every right to believe that the refusal of the arms of Achilles was an act of *hybris* and he would be justified in feeling both anger and dishonour.

[24] See above n.6

[25] Sophocles, *Ajax*, 41. 'χόλῳ βαρυνθεὶς τῶν Ἀχιλλείων ὅπλων'. Translations adapted from P. J. Finglass, *Sophocles: Ajax*. (Cambridge: Cambridge University Press, 2011).

[26] Sophocles, *Ajax*, 23. 'ὥστ᾽ οὔποτ᾽ Αἴανθ᾽ οἵδ᾽ **ἀτιμάσουσ᾽** ἔτι'.

[27] Sophocles, *Ajax*, 442–44, 'εἰ ζῶν Ἀχιλλεὺς τῶν ὅπλων τῶν ὧν πέρι κρίνειν ἔμελλε κράτος ἀριστείας τινί, οὐκ ἄν τις αὔτ᾽ ἔμαρψεν ἄλλος ἀντ᾽ ἐμοῦ'.

MacDowell notes that *hybris* can be the act of taking from someone something that belongs to them, as well as denying someone something that they are owed.[28] He quotes the exchange between Agamemnon and Achilles in the *Iliad* as the first case of *hybris* seen in Greek literature: When Agamemnon deprives Achilles of his prize of war (Briseis), something he was owed, he deprives Achilles of his honour *and* Achilles is furious at this insult.[29] Fisher picks this up and develops this concept of *hybris* being linked to dishonour, noting that if someone commits *hybris* against another, it shows that they do not value or honour them, and it can cause shame and lead to the subject feeling angry and yearning for revenge. He argues that injured honour is at the heart of almost all instances of hybris.[30] He uses as a contextual example, Demosthenes (21.71) in which Demosthenes notes that 'it was not the blow that inspired his anger, it was the dishonour; it is not being beaten that is terrible for free men, terrible though it is, it is being beaten in *hybris*'. As will become evident, Ajax indeed follows this pattern of being angry and having a feeling of dishonour and later shame, which Fisher notes is inherent in men who have been victim to an act of *hybris*.

Hybris is characteristic of tragic heroes, and is often displayed by mortals through an expression of excessive pride and met with punishment by the gods.[31] Sophocles is clearly using this formula when he inserts the hybristic words of Ajax telling Athena that he needs no help on the battlefield.[32] These words would demonstrate excessive pride and

[28] D.M. MacDowell, '"Hybris" in Athens', *Greece & Rome* 23.1, 1976, 14–31, p. 19.

[29] *Iliad* 1. 190; B.M.W. Knox, 'The Ajax of Sophocles', *Harvard Studies in Classical Philology* 65, 1961, 1–37, compares the experiences of Achilles and Ajax esp pp. 51–2.

[30] N.R.E. Fisher, 'Hybris' and Dishonour: I', *Greece and Rome* 23.2, 1976, 177–93, p. 180.

[31] N.R.E. Fisher, 'Hybris' and Dishonour: II', *Greece and Rome* 26.1, 1979, 32–47, p. 32.

[32] Sophocles, *Ajax*, 774. Sophocles has made three key decisions in his adaptation of the Ajax myth, he has included hybristic remarks from Ajax insisting he needs no assistance from Athena during the Trojan war (Sophocles, *Ajax*, 774–75), which appear to be innovation on his own part. Sophocles also makes it clear that the decision to award the arms to Odysseus was made by the Greek commanders (Sophocles, *Ajax*, 445), and lastly, he has included an attack on the commanders/livestock. The introduction of the hybristic remarks lays the foundations for an individualistic, arrogant Ajax and the award of the arms being decided by the generals gives Ajax the opportunity to commit the ultimate military hybris in attempting to murder his generals and friends, an act that the Homeric Ajax simply would not have been capable of.

would suggest that Ajax believes that he does not require assistance from the gods. Blundell argues that Ajax's character is in contrast to Odysseus, who acts with caution and demonstrates *sophrosune* (the ancient Greek concept of soundness of mind).[33] Odysseus shows respect for authority, for example, while he does not wish to see the mad Ajax, he submits and does as Athena says.[34] Odysseus also recognises his place as a mortal.[35] Ajax on the other hand, does not recognise authority (he attempts to murder his superiors) or his limitations as a mortal (he claims he does not need the assistance of Athena on the battlefield). Blundell recognises that Ajax's emotional reaction and violent revenge resembles that of a Homeric god. This can be seen in the contemplations of the chorus when they deliberate who could have sent Ajax mad. The Chorus ask whether it could be Artemis; because she was not honoured after success.[36] Or perhaps it was Ares, who tried to avenge a dishonouring (λώβαν) by undertaking a night-time plan.[37] Both of these explanations: being angry because you were not honoured after a success, and avenging a dishonouring in the night mirror Ajax's emotional response and retaliation highlighting the extremity of his reaction.

Menalaus also labels Ajax hybristic when the Greeks consider what must be done with his body. Menelaus states: 'Previously he was the hybristic one, now it is my turn to think big'.[38] It is clear then, that Sophocles made his Ajax a hybristic hero, he would have been recognised as such by the audience and was labelled as such by Menelaus within the play. This is further emphasised by Cairns, who notes that the chorus immediately shut down Menelaus, telling him not to be hybristic (ὑβριστὴς) over the dead man.[39] Cairns suggests that once Menelaus speaks of it being his turn to 'think big' that the audience would be

[33] M.W. Blundell, *Helping Friends and Harming Enemies: A Study in Sophocles and Greek Ethics* (Cambridge: Cambridge University Press, 1989), p. 64.

[34] Sophocles, *Ajax,* 88.

[35] Sophocles, *Ajax*, 125–26.

[36] Sophocles, *Ajax*, 172–76.

[37] Sophocles, *Ajax*, 179–81.

[38] Sophocles, *Ajax*,1087–88. 'ἕρπει παραλλὰξ ταῦτα. πρόσθεν οὗτος ἦν αἴθων **ὑβριστής**, νῦν δ᾽ ἐγὼ **μέγ᾽ αὖ φρονῶ**'.

[39] D. Cairns, 'Hybris, Dishonour, and Thinking Big', *The Journal of Hellenic Studies* 116, 1996, 1–32.

alarmed and know this was hybristic and not the right state of mind, which is confirmed by the chorus leader's remarks.

So, it is evident that Ajax is angry due to the loss of the arms, which he sees as a dishonour and an act of *hybris* against him. This leads Ajax to undertake a night-time mission in which he plans to murder the Greek generals for the dishonour they have served him. We have two accounts of Ajax's actions, first by Athena who tells Odysseus that Ajax hacked, cleaved spines, and bound and whipped what he believed to be the ancient Greek commanders: 'There he fell upon the horned beasts and killed many by hacking them, cleaving spines all around him'.[40] The use of 'phonos' when referring to the killing of animals has an unusually strong negative colouring.[41] It is essentially a murdering or torturing, it is a violent slaughter. The use of K's and X's was also a common technique used to make the sentence sound harsher.[42] Tecmessa adds:

> And some he cut through the neck, while others he turned on their backs, cut their throats, and hacked through their spines; while others he tortured while bound as if they were men, in his onslaughts on the flocks.[43]

The variety of verbs used to describe Ajax's violence is a deliberate attempt to convey the intensity of the violence.[44] There is a strong emphasis on this not being a conventional use of the sword, it is a torturing. On top of this, Ajax tells Athena that he intends to tie Odysseus to a pillar and whip him to death.[45] This would have been recognised by the audience as an unacceptable form of violence.[46] Athena immediately rebukes Ajax and says: 'Now don't torture the poor man like that'.[47] Athena does not tell Ajax to supress his violence, but simply not to torture Odysseus in this way, binding and whipping was more commonly known

[40] Sophocles, *Ajax*, 55. 'ἔνθ' εἰσπεσὼν ἔκειρε πολύκερων φόνον κύκλῳ ῥαχίζων'.

[41] Finglass, Sophocles *Ajax*, 154.

[42] W.B. Stanford, *Sophocles Ajax* (London: Macmillan, 1963).

[43] Sophocles, *Ajax*, 298–300. 'καὶ τοὺς μὲν ηὐχένιζε, τοὺς δ' ἄνω τρέπων ἔσφαζε κἀρράχιζε, τοὺς δὲ δεσμίους ᾐκίζεθ' ὥστε φῶτας ἐν ποίμναις πίτνων'.

[44] Finglass, Sophocles *Ajax*, 228.

[45] Sophocles, *Ajax*, 108–10.

[46] Cf. (Aeschines 1.59) (Herodotus 1.114–5).

[47] Sophocles, *Ajax*, 111. 'μὴ δῆτα τὸν δύστηνον ὧδέ γ' αἰκίσῃ'.

as a punishment for a slave.[48] Within the play, Odysseus is clear in his denunciation of Ajax's actions. Odysseus labels the act incomprehensible (ἄσκοπον).[49] Odysseus also asks: 'What was this daring and boldness of mind with which he acted?'[50] Finglass argues that the datives convey 'amazement and disapproval'.[51] So it is clear that Odysseus, who represents the wise soldier, is utterly astonished that Ajax would attempt to murder his generals in the middle of the night.

McHardy argues that a loss of honour could spark an angry counter-attack by a man looking to restore his honour. However, revenge was not necessarily an automatic response, men would calculate and weigh up their options before deciding if an act of revenge would be worthwhile.[52] Ajax's reaction is driven by emotion and dishonour, but it is also calculated, so one must ask why he risked murdering the Greeks in order to take the arms of Achilles. McHardy argues that 'the connection between success as a warrior and social status was equally pronounced for the classical Greeks as for Homeric heroes'.[53] The arms were made by a god and would have been a huge symbol of military strength, in a culture where social status was linked to military success, it would be understandable for a man to risk his life for this type of item. Therefore, while Ajax's mission is often seen as representative of a Homeric past,[54] striving for honour and its links to military success were still alive by the time *Ajax* would have been performed (442 BC).[55] The initial response and lengths

48 Finglass, Sophocles *Ajax*, 168.

49 Finglass, Sophocles *Ajax*, 143; I. L. F. De Jong, 'Where Narratology Meets Stylistics: The Seven Versions of Ajax's Madness', in I.J.F. De Jong and A. Rijksbaron (eds), *Sophocles and the Greek Language: Aspects of Diction, Syntax and Pragmatics* (Leiden: Brill, 2006), p. 77 n. 12 translates it as 'the deed is such as no one would have expected beforehand'.

50 Sophocles, *Ajax*, *46*. 'ποίαισι τόλμαις ταῖσδε καὶ φρενῶν θράσει'.

51 Finglass, Sophocles *Ajax* 152.

52 F. McHardy, *Revenge in Athenian Culture* (London: Gerald Duckworth and Co. Ltd, 2008), pp. 1–7.

53 Ibid., p. 94.

54 Knox, 'The Ajax of Sophocles'; Simpson, 'Sophocles' Ajax'; Winnington-Ingram, *Sophocles*; C. Segal, *Tragedy and Civilisation: An Interpretation of Sophocles* (Cambridge, MA: Harvard University Press, 1981).

55 See e.g. Leionidas (Herodotus 7.220.f), Nicias (Thucydides 7.48.4), Anaxibius (Xenophon Hell IV 8.39). See also the contrasting fates of Aristodemus and Eurytus (Herodotus 7.228ff).

to which Ajax goes to regain his honour would have been recognisable to the audience,[56] even if seen as extreme and undesirable.

After being dishonoured, Ajax was overcome by rage, which led him to commit a violent act of military hybris, following this attack Ajax is overwhelmed with pain, grief, and shame. We get an insight into Ajax's emotional state through Tecmessa, Tecmessa claims:

> And now, in his sanity, he has fresh pain. For to behold self-inflicted sufferings, when no one else has contributed to them, lays sharp pangs to the soul.[57]

As Finglass highlights, the pain is to the soul and described as self-inflicted and that no one else has contributed to it—it is very much an internal grief.[58] This is an important distinction made by Tecmessa, she seems here to be placing the blame on Ajax, and claiming that his pain is from within, it is a personal pain inflicted from his loss of honour after losing out on Achilles arms. The chorus also confirms that Ajax's pain originated from the loss of the arms: 'So that time was the potent source of sorrows, when a contest of valour was established for the arms'.[59] Tecmessa then addresses his madness: But now that he has relief and respite from his sickness, he is totally racked with painful grief, and we likewise, no less than before.[60]

This is a common reaction following an attack of madness,[61] Ajax is now no longer sick (mad) as Tecmessa realises, but he is now suffering with grief following the actions he committed when he was insane. Therefore, Tecmessa's response demonstrates that Ajax is suffering from two different pains which have two different causes, one internal (the loss of

[56] See Isocrates 20.5–6: where 'aikeia' and 'atimia' are involved, men have every right to be angry.

[57] Sophocles, *Ajax*, 259–62. 'καὶ νῦν φρόνιμος νέον ἄλγος ἔχει: τὸ γὰρ ἐσλεύσσειν οἰκεῖα πάθη, μηδενὸς ἄλλου παραπράξαντος, μεγάλας ὀδύνας ὑποτείνει'.

[58] Finglass, Sophocles *Ajax* 217.

[59] Sophocles, *Ajax*, 934–36. 'μέγας ἄρ' ἦν ἐκεῖνος ἄρχων χρόνος πημάτων, ἦμος ἀριστόχειρ … ὅπλων ἔκειτ' ἀγὼν πέρι'.

[60] Sophocles, *Ajax*, 274–76. 'νῦν δ' ὡς ἔληξε κἀνέπνευσε τῆς νόσου, κεῖνός τε λύπῃ πᾶς ἐλήλαται κακῇ ἡμεῖς θ' ὁμοίως οὐδὲν ἧσσον ἢ πάρος'.

[61] Cf. Euripides (Herakles 1229–1241), Euripides (Orestes 394–400), Euripides (Bacchae 1280–1290).

honour from the denial of the arms and not being able to take revenge) and one external (madness sent by Athena which made him butcher animals, which is cowardly and humiliating). Tecmessa tells us: 'But now, laid low by this evil fate, the man sits quietly where he has fallen, without food, without drink, in the midst of beasts slain by the sword'.[62] The refusal of food and drink is a common sign of trauma in Greek tragedy,[63] and a character sitting down in tragedy can be a sign of grief. The refusal of food and drink as well as the lack of physical movement builds towards the representation of Ajax as a corpse.[64]

Ajax's shame derives from his fear of mockery and laughter from the Greeks. Ajax proclaims: 'Alas for their laughter! What a **hybris**, it seems, I have suffered!'[65] Further, he states: 'I suppose you laugh long and loud in your delight',[66] and later: 'And they have escaped, against my will, and are laughing'.[67] The first mention of the concept of laughing at your enemies is introduced by Athena: 'Well, isn't laughing at enemies the sweetest form of laughter'.[68] Athena goads Odysseus into laughing at the mad Ajax, because he attempted to kill him, but failed, but Odysseus does not take the bait, something that cannot be said of Ajax, as Tecmessa tells us:

> Some against the Atridae, some concerning Odysseus, laughing loudly at the extent of the violent vengeance inflicted on them in his raid.[69]

When Ajax believes he has killed the Greeks and has Odysseus bound to a pillar, he laughed loudly. This further demonstrates the idea that Athena and Ajax share similar philosophies, and both adhere to the concept of 'help friends and harm enemies'. Ajax laughed when he believed he had

[62] Sophocles, *Ajax*, 313–35. 'νῦν δ' ἐν τοιᾷδε κείμενος κακῇ τύχῃ ἄσιτος ἀνήρ, ἄποτος, ἐν μέσοις βοτοῖς σιδηροκμῆσιν ἥσυχος θακεῖ πεσών'.

[63] Finglass, Sophocles *Ajax* 233.

[64] Ibid., 233.

[65] Sophocles, *Ajax*, 367. 'ὤμοι γέλωτος, οἷον **ὑβρίσθην** ἄρα'.

[66] Sophocles, *Ajax*, 382. 'ἦ που πολὺν γέλωθ' ὑφ' ἡδονῆς ἄγεις'.

[67] Sophocles, *Ajax*, 454–55. 'κεῖνοι δ' ἐπεγγελῶσιν ἐκπεφευγότες, ἐμοῦ μὲν οὐχ ἑκόντος'.

[68] Sophocles, *Ajax*, 79. 'οὔκουν γέλως ἥδιστος εἰς ἐχθροὺς γελᾶν'.

[69] Sophocles, *Ajax*, 302–4. 'τοὺς δ' ἀμφ' Ὀδυσσεῖ, συντιθεὶς γέλων πολύν, ὅσην κατ' αὐτῶν ὕβριν ἐκτίσαιτ' ἰών'.

the power, so it was only right for him to expect the laughter of the Greeks when he failed, because he would have (and did) laugh himself. Moreover, Ajax is ashamed to face his father following his actions. Ajax proclaims: 'And when I appear how will I show my face to my father, Telamon?'[70] Ajax asks: 'How ever will he bring himself to look upon me, when I appear naked, bereft of those prizes which he won as a great crown of glory'.[71]

This fear of looking a father in the eye is a typical *aidos* reaction linked to the idea that fathers hope that their sons will be greater warriors than themselves and preserve family honour.[72] These undertones are seen in the mirroring of Ajax's scene with his son Eurysaces with Hector and his son Astyanax (Iliad 6.479). Ajax, uses the word *γυμνὸν* and although he is not literally naked, the use of this word evokes shame, as Ajax believes that without the arms of Achilles, he is naked.[73] In addition, Ajax highlighting the fact that Telamon won his glory and reaped the rewards for doing so highlights the idea that for him, the recognition of his glory is just as important if not more important than his actual achievements at war. His idea of self-worth is completely framed by concepts of honour and shame. It is precisely this mindset which creates a vulnerability to trauma when military honour is not achieved. He goes on to suggest that this kind of shame cannot be endured.

After deciding he cannot endure a life without honour, Ajax decides to take his own life. He cries: 'Io darkness, my light, o Erebus, most bright for me. Take, take me as your inhabitant, take me!'[74] This is in contrast to the Homeric Ajax who calls for light for guidance when mist shrouds the battlefield (Iliad 17.645–7), and also mirrors Athena darkening the eyes of Ajax when Odysseus comes to his tent. The fact that Ajax calls for darkness, and calls it his light, and describes the underworld as the most bright for him, stresses how his mindset is at odds with conventional ideas

[70] Sophocles, *Ajax*, 462–63. 'καὶ ποῖον ὄμμα πατρὶ δηλώσω φανεὶς Τελαμῶνι'.

[71] Sophocles, *Ajax*, 463–65. 'πῶς με τλήσεταί ποτ' εἰσιδεῖν γυμνὸν φανέντα τῶν ἀριστείων ἄτερ, ὧν αὐτὸς ἔσχε στέφανον εὐκλείας μέγαν'.

[72] Cairns, *Aidos*, 231. A feeling of shame and a wish not to look loved ones in the eye can also be a reaction to tragic madness, see both Herakles (Herakles 1231–33) and Agave (Bacchae 1381–87).

[73] Cairns, *Aidos*, 273.

[74] Sophocles, *Ajax*, 394–98. 'ἰὼ σκότος, ἐμὸν φάος, ἔρεβος ὦ φαεννότατον, ὡς ἐμοί, ἕλεσθ' ἕλεσθέ μ' οἰκήτορα, ἕλεσθέ μ.

of fifth-century Athens.[75] Ajax then contemplates whether dying in battle would be an honourable end for him, but decides that this would give the Greeks too much satisfaction, Ajax says: 'This cannot be. Some enterprise must be sought from which I may show my aged father that I, his son, am no coward'.[76] Finally, Ajax decides: 'But the noble man must either live well or die well'.[77] Ajax is searching for a death that will restore the most honour possible, and he decides that a glorious death would be better than living on in shame.[78]

There is debate among scholars as to whether Ajax takes his own life due to shame, or as one final act of revenge against the Greeks. Van Hoof argues that Ajax had to take his own life after the disgrace he had faced, he concludes: 'where modern observers would rather assume despair or grief as the predominant motive the ancient reporter was inclined to put shame in the fore-front'.[79] On the other hand, Burnett argues that 'Ajax does not merely destroy himself in the final scene; he also curses, and his curse transforms his death into a renewed revenge'.[80] Further, Burnett highlights that this suicidal revenge curse could be seen as heroic and admired in classical Greece and this transforms Ajax's death into a noble one rather than a shameful one.[81] I believe both can be true, at no point does Ajax indicate that he feels remorse for attempting to murder the Greek generals and as his passing words demonstrate, he explicitly still wants them dead. However, I believe it is his shame regarding his lost honour which leads him to take this drastic action. He wants to die because he cannot face his father and the humiliation and laughter of his enemies, but he also wants his death to be heroic so that he can regain as much honour as possible. On top of this, Ajax wants the Greeks to pay, they committed

[75] Cairns, *Aidos*, 255.

[76] Sophocles, *Ajax*, 466–69, 470–72. 'οὐκ ἔστι ταῦτα. πεῖρά τις ζητητέα τοιάδ' ἀφ' ἧς γέροντι δηλώσω πατρὶ μή τοι φύσιν γ' ἄσπλαγχνος ἐκ κείνου γεγώς'.

[77] 'Sophocles, Ajax, 479–80. 'ἀλλ' ἢ καλῶς ζῆν ἢ καλῶς τεθνηκέναι τὸν εὐγενῆ χρή'.

[78] Again, this is an experience that both Achilles and Herakles are faced with and both express a desire for death over living a life without honour and glory. Also, see above n.55 for instances of soldiers wishing to die a glorious death in battle as appose to living.

[79] A.J.L. Van Hoof, *From Autothanasia to Suicide: Self Killing in Classical Antiquity* (London: Routledge, 1990), 120.

[80] A.P. Burnett, *Revenge in Attic and Later Tragedy* (London and Berkeley: University of California Press, 1998), 86.

[81] Ibid., 93.

a *hybris* against him and took what was rightly his. Therefore, taking his life while cursing the Greeks is his only available option to accomplish all three of his desires. There are examples of soldiers taking their lives due to shame or for a lack of honour throughout Herodotus, for example, Pantites who hangs himself in dishonour once he returned to Sparta,[82] or Othrades who Herodotus tells us killed himself from shame returning to Sparta as a survivor.[83] It is clear that being overcome by shame and feeling dishonoured were reasons for men to take their own lives in fifth-century Greece.

Sumio Yoshitake tackles when it was acceptable for an ancient Greek hero to take his own life and concludes that shame, despair, disgrace, and hopelessness were motives that could justify a man taking his own life.[84] Regarding honour, Yoshitake highlights that Herakles longed for suicide, until Theseus arrived and promised him a recovery of his honour.[85] Once Theseus had made this offer, it would have been unacceptable for him to take his own life, as he would not have been taking it out of a hopeless loss of honour, but rather out of pain. We see these sentiments in Aristotle's *Nicomachean Ethics*: 'But to seek death in order to escape from poverty, or the pangs of love, or from pain or sorrow, is not the act of a courageous man, but rather of a coward'.[86] Furthermore, Yoshitake comments on the role of the divine, he notes that suicide is not normal behaviour when a man is under divine protection, but it becomes permissible when he has been forsaken by the gods'.[87] As is evident in this play, Athena (the usual guardian of warriors) has turned against Ajax. Socrates, in a conversation with Cebes in Plato's *Phaedo*, seems to articulate this view. He tells Cebes that:

> The gods are our guardians and that we men are one of the chattels of the gods... if one of your chattels should kill itself when you had not indicated that you wished it to die, would you be angry with it and punish it if

[82] Herodotus 7.232.

[83] Herodotus 1.82.

[84] S. Yoshitake, 'Disgrace, Grief and Other Ills: Herakles' Rejection of Suicide', *The Journal of Hellenic Studies* 114, 1994, 138–39.

[85] Ibid., 144.

[86] Nic. Eth. 1116a.1.

[87] Yoshitake, 'Disgrace', 148.

> you could? Then perhaps from this point of view it is not unreasonable to say that a man must not kill himself until god sends some necessity upon him.[88]

In conclusion, Yoshitake notes that Sophocles was aware of the fact that suicide was a way to preserve honour, and because of this, he has key characters take their own life 'in such a way that their suicides appear to be splendid achievements that might restore their honour and remedy their ills at the same time'.[89] It appears evident that the steps leading to Ajax's decision to take his own life were contextually understandable: Greeks of the fifth century could take their own life to preserve honour, and this often happened when the prospect of living was hopeless and the subject had been abandoned by the gods. The way in which he kills himself (replicating a kill in battle with his enemy's sword), as well as uttering a curse to his enemies was also comprehensible and a sign of noble honour to the audience and they would have understood that Ajax's only option was to take his own life.

Overall, the script-based methodology has identified the full complexity of Ajax's emotional experience within its cultural context. Ajax is a man who loses his honour when he is not awarded the arms of Achilles and is traumatised. This trauma leads to his retaliation by attempting to murder the Greeks by night. Although the ancient Greeks did not view Ajax's reaction as 'traumatic' or describe it as such, fifth-century Athenian society, with its fixation on honour, and honour being directly related to military success bred these situations and experiences that led men to go to great lengths in order to preserve their honour. The reaction of Ajax would have been recognised as excessive, hybristic, and unacceptable by the audience. So although the Greeks did not have a concept of 'combat trauma' per se, they were aware that men could wreak havoc in an attempt to preserve their honour, and that this was a danger to their society. At every turn, Ajax's emotional responses are comprehensible within their historical context, how he processes these emotions and chooses to react demonstrate his trauma. For a man to turn on his allies and attempt to murder them, and eventually kill himself in order to preserve a degree of honour demonstrates that in some cases this obsession with honour could be debilitating for ancient Greek warriors of the fifth-century.

[88] Phaedo 62b–62c.

[89] Yoshitake, 'Disgrace', 150.

Bibliography

Allen, D.S., *The World of Prometheus: The Politics of Punishing in Democratic Athens* (Princeton: Princeton University Press, 2000).

Blundell, M.W., *Helping Friends and Harming Enemies: A Study in Sophocles and Greek Ethics* (Cambridge: Cambridge University Press, 1989).

Braund, S. and Most, G.W., *Ancient Anger, Perspectives from Homer to Galen* (Cambridge: Cambridge University Press, 2003).

Brouwers, J., *Ancient Warfare IX.4* (Rotterdam: Karwansaray Publishers, 2013).

Burnett, A.P., *Revenge in Attic and Later Tragedy* (London and Berkeley: University of California Press, 1998).

Cairns, D. and Fulkerson, L., *Emotions Between Greece and Rome* (London: Institute of Classical Studies, 2015).

Cairns, D., 'Look Both Ways: Studying Emotion in Ancient Greece', *Critical Quarterly* 50.4, 2008, 43–62.

Carins, D., 'Hybris, Dishonour, and Thinking Big', *The Journal of Hellenic Studies* 116, 1996, 1-32.

Cairns, D., *Aidos, the Psychology and Ethics of Honour and Shame in Ancient Greek Literature* (Oxford: Clarendon Press, 1993).

Caston, V. and Weineck, S-M., *Our Ancient Wars: Rethinking War through the Classics* (Ann Arbor, MI.: University of Michigan Press, 2016).

Chaniotis A., *Unveiling Emotions. Sources and Methods for the Study of Emotions in the Greek World* (Stuttgart: Franz Steiner Verlog, 2012).

Cohen, D., 'The Imagery of Sophocles: A Study of Ajax's Suicide', *Greece and Rome* 25.1, 1978, 24–36.

Cole, E., 'Post-Traumatic Stress Disorder and the Performance Reception of Sophocles' *Ajax*', in D..Stuttard (ed), *Looking at Ajax* (London: Bloomsbury, 2019), pp. 151–160.

Crowley, J., *The Psychology of the Athenian Hoplite: The culture of Combat in Classical Athens* (Cambridge: Cambridge University Press, 2012).

Crowley, J., Beyond the Universal Soldier: Combat Trauma in Classical Antiquity', in P. Meineck and D. Konstan (eds), *Combat Trauma and the Ancient Greeks*. (London: Palgrave, 2014), pp. 105–130.

Crowley, J. and Rees, O., 'PTSD in Ancient Greece: Was there mental trauma in ancient warfare?', in J. Brouwers (ed), *Ancient Warfare IX.4* (Rotterdam: Karwansaray Publishers, 2013).

De Jong, I. L. F., 'Where Narratology Meets Stylistics: The Seven Versions of Ajax's Madness', in I.J.F. De Jong and A. Rijksbaron (eds), *Sophocles and the Greek Language: Aspects of Diction, Syntax and Pragmatics* (Leiden: Brill, 2006), pp. 73–94.

Doerries, B., *The Theater of War: What Ancient Greek Tragedies Can Teach Us Today.* (New York: Knopf, 2015).

Finglass, P.J., *Sophocles: Ajax.* (Cambridge: Cambridge University Press, 2011).

Fisher, N., 'Violence, Masculinity and the law in Classical Athens', in L. Foxhall and J. Salmon (eds), *When men were men: Masculinity, Power and Identity in Classical Antiquity* (London: Routledge, 1998), pp. 68–97.

Fisher, N.R.E., *Hybris: A Study in the Values of Honour and Shame in Ancient Greece.* (Warminster: Aris and Phillips, 1992).

Fisher, N.R.E., 'Hybris' and Dishonour: II', *Greece and Rome* 26.1, 1979, 32–47

Fisher, N.R.E., 'Hybris' and Dishonour: I', *Greece and Rome* 23.2, 1976, 77–193.

Gasti, H., 'Sophocles' "Ajax": The Military "Hybris"', *Quaderni Urbinati di Cultura Classica* 40.1, 1992, 81–93.

Harris, V.W., *Restraining Rage, The Ideology of Anger Control in Classical Antiquity* (Cambridge, MA: Harvard University Press, 2001)

Hesk. J., *Sophocles: Ajax* (London: Duckworth, 2003).

Harris, V.W., (ed) *Mental Disorders in the Classical World* (Leiden: Brill, 2013).

Herman, G., *Morality and Behaviour in Democratic Athens: A Social History* (Cambridge: Cambridge University Press, 2006).

Holmes, B., *The Symptom and the Subject: The Emergence of the Physical Body in Ancient Greece* (Princeton: Princeton University Press, 2010).

Kaster, R.A., *Emotion, Restraint and Community in Ancient Rome* (Oxford: Oxford University Press, 2005).

Katsouris, A.G., 'The suicide motif in Ancient Drama', *Dioniso. Di studi sul teatro antico* 47, 1976, 5–37.

Kennedy, R.F., *Athena's Justice: Athena, Athens and the Concept of Justice in Greek Tragedy* (New York: Peter Lang, 2009).

Knox, B.M.W., *The Heroic Temper: Studies in Sophoclean Tragedy* (Berkeley: University of California Press, 1964).

Knox, B.M.W., 'The Ajax of Sophocles', *Harvard Studies in Classical Philology* 65, 1961, 1–37.

Konstan, D., *The Emotions of the Ancient Greeks: Studies in Aristotle and Classical Literature* (Toronto: University of Toronto Press, 2006).

Lawrence, S., 'Ancient Ethics, the Heroic Code, and the Morality of Sophocles' *Ajax*', *Greece & Rome* 52.1, 2005, 18–33.

MacDowell, D.M., '"Hybris" in Athens', *Greece & Rome* 23.1, 1976, 14–31.

McHardy, F., *Revenge in Athenian Culture* (London: Gerald Duckworth and Co. Ltd, 2008).

Meineck, P. and Konstan, D. (eds), *Combat Trauma and the Ancient Greeks* (London: Palgrave, 2014).

Obrien-Moore, A., *Madness in Ancient Literature* (Weimar: R. Wahner Sohn, 1924).

Padel, R., *Whom Gods Destroy: Elements of Greek and Tragic Madness* (Princeton: Princeton University Press, 1995).

Padel, R., *In and Out of the Mind: Greek Images of the Tragic Self* (Princeton: Princeton University Press, 1994).
Pegler, J., *Curing Madness* (London: Chipmunka Publishing, 2011).
Sanders, E., *Envy and Jealousy in Classical Greece: A Socio-Psychological Approach* (Oxford: Oxford University Press, 2014).
Segal, C., *Tragedy and Civilisation: An Interpretation of Sophocles* (Cambridge, MA: Harvard University Press, 1981)
Shay, J., *Achilles in Vietnam, Combat Trauma and the Undoing of Character* (New York: Pocket Books, 1994).
Shay, J., *Odysseus in America. Combat Trauma and the Trials of Homecoming* (New York: Scribner, 2003).
Simon, B., *Mind and Madness in Ancient Greece: The Classical Roots in Modern Psychiatry* (Ithaca: Cornell University Press, 1978).
Simpson, M., 'Sophocles Ajax: His Madness and Transformation', *Arethusa* 2.1, 1969, 88–103.
Stanford, W.B., *Sophocles Ajax* (London: Macmillan, 1963).
Thiher, A., *Revels in Madness: Insanity in Medicine and Literature* (Ann Arbor: University of Michigan Press, 1999).
Thumiger, C., 'Mental Insanity in the Hippocratic texts: A Pragmatic Perspective', *Mnemosyne: A Journal of Classical Studies* 68.2, 2015, 210–234.
Thumiger, C., *Hidden Paths, Self and Characterisation in Greek Tragedy: Euripides Bacchae* (London: Institute of Classical Studies, 2007).
Tritle, L.A., *From Melos to My Lai, War and Survival* (London: Routledge, 2000).
Tritle, L.A. '"Ravished Minds" in the Ancient World', in P . Meineck and D. Konstan (eds), *Combat Trauma and the Ancient Greeks*. (London: Palgrave, 2014), pp. 87–104.
Ustinova, Y. and Cardena, E., 'Combat Stress Disorders and Their Treatment in Ancient Greece' *Psychological Trauma: Theory, Research, Practice, and Policy* June.2, 2014, 1–10.
Van Hoof, A.J.L., *From Autothanasia to suicide: Self Killing in Classical Antiquity* (London: Routledge, 1990).
Wertenbaker, T. *Our Ajax* (London: Faber & Faber, 2013).
Winkler, J.J. and Zeitlin, F.I., *Nothing to do with Dionysus? Athenian Drama in its social context* (Princeton: Princeton University Press, 1990).
Winnington-Ingram, R.P., *Sophocles: An Interpretation* (Cambridge: Cambridge University Press, 1980).
Yoshitake, S., Disgrace, Grief and Other Ills: Herakles' Rejection of Suicide', *The Journal of Hellenic Studies* 114, 1994, 135–153.

Legal Evidence for Roman PTSD?

Andrew Fear

Since the invention of its diagnosis in 1980,[1] there has been considerable academic interest in attempting to find traces of PTSD in troops serving before the modern era. The majority of this interest has focussed on the ancient Greek world, not least because of Jonathon Shay's groundbreaking study *Achilles in Vietnam*. However, the longest lasting professional army in the ancient world was to be found not in Greece, but at Rome, where standing, professional troops were a feature of society for almost half a millennium.[2] While no ancient institution is as well-documented as those of the modern era, this longevity generated a considerable amount of material which means that the Roman army

[1] A. Howell, 'The Demise of PTSD: From Governing Through Trauma to Governing Resilience', *Alternatives* 37.3, 2012, 214–26.

[2] Roughly from the 'Marian reforms' of the early first century BC to the collapse of the Western Empire in AD 476. The Eastern Roman Empire lies outside the scope of this paper.

A. Fear (✉)
University of Manchester, Manchester, UK
e-mail: andrew.fear@manchester.ac.uk

O. Rees et al. (eds.), *Combat Stress in Pre-modern Europe*, Mental Health in Historical Perspective,
https://doi.org/10.1007/978-3-031-09947-2_5

is now by far the best attested and understood military force from antiquity. Despite this, tracing PTSD in the Imperial Roman period has proved more difficult than isolating a will o' the wisp. In his *Acts of War*, Richard Holmes confidently asserts that 'there is reason to doubt' that PTSD is a product of twentieth-century warfare, but, faced with the paucity of evidence, almost immediately concedes that 'Psychiatric casualties were undoubtedly relatively uncommon prior to the twentieth century'.[3] As good British empiricists, we must agree with David Hume that an 'is' cannot be deduced from an 'ought', so how then are we to proceed? Our problem is threefold. First, there is the protean nature of the diagnosis itself which is continually changing. Second, is the question as to whether this modern diagnosis can justifiably be applied to a very different period of time which arguably possessed a radically different outlook on the world from that found in present-day Europe. Third, is the nature and quality of contemporary evidence from the period under consideration.

It must be the case that to assert PTSD was present in antiquity, we need clear testimonia that a substantial number of individuals were so afflicted. Mankind is composed of individuals who react to the same circumstances in a multiplicity of ways. It would be equally rash either to assert that such a phenomenon never existed for anyone in antiquity or to rush to generalise from one individual's experience to Roman society as a whole. Thus to show that PTSD posed a genuine and significant problem for the Roman army, we must demonstrate that substantial numbers of troops exhibited its symptoms. Moreover, we must show that these symptoms were persistent. Recoiling in horror on one occasion does not show the presence of a syndrome, but merely a spontaneous response which may or may not have long-lasting effects. This paper will only deal with the possibility of individuals suffering PTSD. Group combat fatigue is something attested in the modern period and was regarded as highly contagious in the Great War.[4] However, although we have some evidence of mutinies in the Roman army occurring in our period, our descriptions of them imply that they had nothing to do with combat, but were rather focussed on grievances concerning pay, conditions of service, and

[3] R. Holmes, *Acts of War: the Behaviour of Men in Battle* (London: Cassell, 2003), pp. 255–56.

[4] See Lord Southborough, *Report of the War Office Committee of Enquiry into 'Shell Shock'* (London: HMSO 1922, reprinted 2014), pp. 28–9, 48, 66. For an ancient example of panic spreading through an army, see Caesar, *Bellum Gallicum,* 1.39.

politics.[5] One possible exception occurs early in the reign of Augustus during the Cantabrian wars. According to Dio, Agrippa 'marched against the Cantabrians, but had some trouble with his troops as not a few of them were too old for service and had been worn down by the continual strain (συνεχείᾳ) of the wars. They feared the Cantabrians as fierce fighters and so did not obey him'.[6] Agrippa's response to this mutiny was to deprive one legion of its honorific title *Augusta* ('the Emperor's own') and here his difficulties seem to have ended. The incident is the nearest we have in the ancient record to evidence for combat fatigue. Rome's campaigns in Cantabria were what would now be called guerrilla warfare which, as can be seen from the US experience in Vietnam, often generates PTSD-related problems. However, other factors may have been at work here. Dio implies that these problematic troops were expecting to be discharged (as had happened during the wars previously fought here in 25 BC) and thus felt that they had 'done their bit'. The reluctance to fight could therefore have been less to do with combat fatigue than with anger at being placed in danger when 'short' to use the common slang of the Vietnam War. This form of 'anxious apprehension' at being placed in danger towards the end of service was a common phenomenon in that war.[7]

To return to potential incidences of PTSD as opposed to combat fatigue, we need to isolate what sort of evidence we need to look for in the ancient record. There are three key elements which regularly feature in diagnoses of PTSD used in modern times and which we can search for in our ancient sources as good signs of problems. These are: 'flashback' dreams or nightmares, continual feelings of insecurity, and depression/suicidal tendencies. If these seem secure markers, our next question is where can they be traced? Any search is hampered by two factors. First, military history did not exist as a genre of writing in antiquity. This is true at all levels. Even the most detailed accounts of warfare which have survived from antiquity, such as Josephus's *Jewish*

[5] L. Fulkerson, *No Regrets: Remorse in Classical Antiquity* (Oxford: Oxford University Press, 2013), pp. 180–85; A. Denman, *An Analysis of Roman Mutiny Narratives through Multiple Perspectives*, Unpublished MA thesis (MacMaster University, 2013).

[6] ἐπ᾽ οὖν τούτους ὁ Ἀγρίππας ἐπιστρατεύσας ἔσχε μέν τι καὶ πρὸς τοὺς στρατιώτας ἔργον: πρεσβύτεροι γὰρ οὐκ ὀλίγοι αὐτῶν ὄντες καὶ τῇ συνεχείᾳ τῶν πολέμων τετρυχωμένοι, τούς τε Καντάβρους ὡς καὶ δυσπολεμήτους δεδιότες, οὐκ ἐπείθοντο αὐτῷ. Dio 54.11.

[7] See P. Bourne, *Men, Stress, and Vietnam* (Boston: Little, Brown, 1970).

War, do not contain the details that we would expect as a standard feature of a modern work. Accounts of battles in our surviving ancient texts are often presented in a highly stylised way where the inclusion of what were deemed appropriate rhetorical patterns takes precedence over recording the details of what in fact happened. Added to this is our second problem: antique writers were disinterested in the experience of the common soldier as opposed to their commanders and it is precisely these former combatants who were most likely to suffer from any form of PTSD. This lack of appetite also appears to be the case with ancient readers who would naturally have been drawn from the higher orders of society. While from the nineteenth century onwards, probably due to the rise of mass democracy and literacy, the memoirs of common soldiers have become increasingly popular with readers, few, if any, appear to have been written in antiquity and none have survived.[8] Our nearest equivalent to this genre appeared in late antiquity in the form of the pseudolives of Dares and Dictys who allegedly fought in the Trojan War. While taken at face value in the medieval period, the original intention of the anonymous authors appears to have been ironic and so they are useless as evidence.[9] Our best surviving non-fictional account is arguably the anonymous *Bellum Hispaniense* which describes Caesar's campaigns in the Iberian peninsula. Its Latinity is extremely poor, and led Rice Holmes notoriously to comment that '*Bellum Hispaniense* is the worst book in Latin literature; and its text is the most deplorable. The language is generally ungrammatical and often unintelligible'. The style of the text led Lord Macaulay to deem it the work of a 'sturdy old centurion who fought better than he wrote', a guess with the text's Loeb editor, A.G. Way,

[8] Thus, there is no ancient equivalent of the plethora of memoirs produced after the Napoleonic Wars. The most famous of these is probably *The Recollections of Rifleman Harris*. Harris, who was illiterate, dictated the book to his friend Capt. Henry Curling, a minor novelist, in the 1830s. The resulting manuscript was then published in 1848. There are very many others, including those written from what in the Roman world would be regarded as the perspective of an 'auxiliary', for example, S. Ram Pande, *From Sepoy to Subedar Being the Life and Adventures of Subedar Sita Ram, a Native Officer of the Bengal Army, Written and Related by Himself*, which was translated from Hindi and published in 1873. The ancient world can offer no equivalents.

[9] For the use of these texts in the Middle Ages, see V. Prosperi, 'The Place of the Father: the Reception of Homer in the Renaissance Canon', in E. Morra (ed), *Building the Canon though the Classics* (Leiden: Brill, 1988), pp. 47–69; and F. Mora-Lebrun, 'Joseph of Exeter: Troy through Dictys and Dares', in Simms, R.C. (ed), *Brill's Companion to Prequels, Sequels, and Retellings of Classical Epic* (Leiden: Brill, 2018), pp. 115–33.

described as 'possibly not far off the truth'.[10] Yet, even this is a matter of dispute and while the *Bellum Hispaniense* indubitably is more honest in its recording of atrocities than Caesar's carefully crafted *Bellum Gallicum,* it still contains very little in the way of soldiers' experience of battle.[11]

Despite these methodological difficulties, sadly the use of ancient evidence in this field has often been somewhat careless. Citations dealing with events hundreds of years apart are concatenated together without caution, and the literary intentions and chronological distance of their authors from their subject matter are also often neglected.[12] We would not use the battle experience of troops from Marlborough's campaigns as evidence for that of soldiers in the Second World War and would be suspicious that a modern writer could easily assume the mental universe of, say, an archer at Agincourt. Yet, similar assumptions are all too readily made when dealing with the many centuries grouped together under the umbrella term of 'antiquity'. The paucity of ancient evidence leads to a temptation to ignore the passage of time in Roman antiquity, but it should be resisted. The role of rhetoric too has been ignored, as has the fact that many of our accounts are written by those with no clear battle experience and substantially after the events they describe. When we look at key authors, these problems are stark. Notoriously Livy's battle narratives are all similar to one another, and Tacitus was described by Theodor Mommsen as 'the most unmilitary of all historians'.[13] Neither are known to have served in the army, and both describe actions at best several generations away from their own time. In Livy's case, many of his battles are set in the distant past, centuries before his own day. Added to these problems is a wish to see poetry or other forms of pure fiction as reliable forms of reportage. This is simply unacceptable. The poets cited are often

[10] T. Rice Holmes, *The Roman Republic and the Founder of the Empire*, vol. 2 (Oxford: Clarendon Press, 1923), p. 298.

[11] The best edition of Caesar's *Bellum Gallicum* is that edited by N. Diourn (1999). A poor prose style is not the preserve of the poor. R.H., Storch, 'The Author Of The "De Bello Hispaniensi": A Cavalry Officer?', *Acta Classica* 20, 1977, 201–04 believes the work to have been written by a cavalry officer, while Van Hoof, 'The Caesar of the "Bellum Hispaniense"', *Mnemosyne,* 27.2, 1974, 123–38 doubts that the work was written by a military man at all.

[12] This is a tendency which at times regrettably mars the otherwise excellent work of Van Lommel.

[13] T. Mommsen, *The Provinces of the Roman Empire: From Caesar to Diocletian,* vol. 1 (London: MacMillan & Co., 1909), p. 181.

ones who appear to have had no experience of battle. A good example is Lucan who provides detailed and grisly accounts of battle in his *Pharsalia* (already events a hundred years in the past when he composed his poem). However, like his equally vivid account of the horrors to be found in druid groves, these are a product of his imagination, not reality. Such material tells us only about reactions to war, either contemporary warfare, though more often in fact warfare in the historical or mythical past, of a small aristocratic group who were normally distanced from the experience of war itself.[14] War poetry written by participants in battle was written at Rome: Naevius wrote an epic on the First Punic War, and Albanovanus Pedo one on his service with Germanicus in Germany in AD 16.[15] However, sadly, of the fragments that remain of these works, none describe battle itself. Moreover, even if they did, problems of literary expectations and autobiographical fallacies would abound. Poetry is not reportage. We would not turn to Lord Tennyson to learn about the experience of soldiers serving in the Crimean War or to GA Henty to learn about the reality of soldiering in the Boer War, though they can tell us about the reactions of their wider society to war, and we must not fall into the same trap when thinking about antiquity.

Added to these problems is that of what our sources do not say. Of what may be called PTSD's 'signature' symptom—'flashback' memories or recurrent nightmares—there is no trace.[16] It is striking, for example, that such dreams do not appear in Artemidorus's *Oneirocritica*, our most sustained discussion of dreams in antiquity. That said, Artemidorus, like Plutarch, has a tendency to dismiss the dreams of the common man as uninteresting and unreliable. Given that it was the common soldier and what would now be styled non-commissioned officers who are most likely to have suffered PTSD, it could be that this silence is not as telling as it at first seems and it is on the common soldier on whom this brief paper

[14] Like Lucan, there is no evidence that Virgil, Statius ever served in the Roman army or had any experience of the empire's frontiers. Horace did fight in the Civil Wars, but there is no trace of PTSD in any of his poetry which treats his participation in battle with light irony, see *Odes* 2.7.10.

[15] Preserved by Seneca, *Suasoriae* 1.15.

[16] Plutarch (*Marius* 45) makes clear that Marius's nightmares when pursued by Sulla at the end of his life are provoked by the imagined future not the past—Marius was suffering from Pre, not Post, Traumatic Stress Disorder.

concentrates. Nevertheless, suspicion is not enough, we need to show why this silence in our sources, if silence it is, is curious.

There are good presumptive reasons to suspect that PTSD was not a common phenomenon in the Imperial Roman period. This was a period characterised by the general brutality of its everyday life, where for most there was a constant presence of death: it was, inter alia, the era of the gladiatorial arena. Moreover, it was an age before the shell. It is not for nothing that 'shell shock' was the common name for what would now be identified as PTSD in the Great War. There is growing evidence that many forms of PTSD have a physical component in the damage done to the brain by concussive explosions.[17] Clearly the Roman soldier was not faced with any similar danger. Shells however also produce psychological stress as shell fire can occur at any time and there is no defence against it. This can engender a constant sense of insecurity and helplessness.[18] A final point which ought not to be forgotten is the sheer volume of noise created by heavy shelling and, again, the prolonged periods of time for which this can be present. There was no equivalent phenomenon in antiquity. Ancient battles were in the main brief affairs, normally lasting 2–3 hours. And within that period, there would be enforced lulls given the physically gruelling nature of hand-to-hand combat.[19] An all-day battle was rare, a two-day one exceptional. In contrast, the battle of the Somme lasted 140 days.[20] Thus for the Roman soldier, unlike his modern counterparts, the experience of battle was short. His enemy was obvious, as was his position. He posed no serious threat beyond the field of battle

[17] S. Baughman Shively, et al., 'Characterisation of Interface Astroglial Scarring in the Human Brain After Blast Exposure: A Post-Mortem Case Series', *The Lancet: Neurology* 15.9, 2016, 944–53.

[18] See S.A. Stouffer, et al., *The American Soldier: Combat and Its Aftermath* (New York: Wiley, 1949). This is a point stressed by Holmes, *Acts of War*, 211, citing a Vietnam veteran, 'I could deal with a man that my talent against his for survival, but how do you deal with him when he ain't even there?'.

[19] See Vegetius, *De Re Militari* 3.9 and A.K. Goldsworthy, *The Roman Army at War, 100 BC-AD 200* (Oxford: Oxford University Press, 1996), pp. 201–06. For lulls in battle, see S. Koon, *Infantry Combat in Livy's Battle Narratives (British Archaeological Reports, International Series 2071)* (Oxford: BAR Publishing, 2010).

[20] Holmes, *Acts of War*, 216, notes that a Napoleonic soldier would have campaigned for years before amassing the same amount of time in combat that troops talking part in the Italian campaign of 1944–1995 accrued. The same is true, perhaps more so, of ancient troops.

and the ability personally to counter his efforts to deal death was clear and constantly available. In the terminology of psychology, this means the Roman soldier maintained an 'internal locus of control', i.e. the belief that he was master of his own fate, as opposed to an 'external locus of control' or the belief that he was at the mercy of forces beyond his control.[21]

While noisy, the sound generated from voices and trumpets reached nothing like the levels produced by modern weapons. Outside of battle, the soldier's life was not stressful. Ranged weapons were few and in general poor, so the constant sense of danger from sniping that pervades many modern military campaigns was simply not present and nor were booby traps, car bombs, and their like. Moreover, the Roman army's practice of operating from fortified bases, normally surrounded by a friendly village, and of building fortified marching camps when on campaign, combined with their enemies' perceived, and actual, inability to overrun such bases, ensured that the Roman soldier slept soundly and securely. Perhaps, we should not neglect either the dominant ideology of the times—that of stoicism. While there was no official belief system in the Roman world, the philosophy of stoicism in a modified populist form provided the assumptions upon which most Romans acted. It held that virtue obtained through reason was sufficient for happiness and that the virtuous man through accepting the ups and downs of the world while preserving his inner virtue could always adapt to his circumstances without losing his internal balance or *eudaimonia*. In the words of Epictetus, the stoic would be 'sick, yet happy; in danger, yet happy; dying, yet happy; in exile and happy; in disgrace and happy'.[22] It would be foolish to believe that all or most Roman soldiers were active believers in this philosophy of self-control, but like Christianity in the West until recently, it was a constant background feature of the Roman soldier's mindset and is likely to have provided a mental defence against despondency that was absent in later periods.[23]

[21] For the 'Locus of Control', see J.B. Rotter, *Social Learning and Clinical Psychology* (Englewood Cliffs, NJ: Prentice-Hall, 1954); R.S., Lazarus and S. Folkman, *Stress, Appraisal, and Coping* (New York: Springer, 1984); and E.J. Peacock and P.T.P. Wong, 'Anticipatory Stress: The Relation of Locus of Control, Optimism, and Control Appraisals to Coping', *Journal of Research In Personality* 30, 1996, 204–22.

[22] Epictetus, Discourses 2.19.

[23] See Seneca, *Epistulae Morales ad Lucilium*, 3.24. For the use of stoicism in a modern military context, see N. Sherman, *Stoic Warriors* (Oxford: Oxford University Press, 2005).

Therefore, as can be seen, reliable contemporary accounts of the Roman soldier are difficult to find. However, one set of ancient evidence perhaps overcomes the objections outlined above. This is that found Roman Law.[24] Legal texts manage to evade many of the difficulties that other forms of literature present for us. They are utilitarian, devoid, in the main, of rhetoric, and were intended to have a direct application to society and thus should mirror its realities. While our main body of Roman Law, Justinian's *Digest*, dates from Late Antiquity, the jurists' opinions and discussions it contains are much earlier in many cases. Among them are a series of rulings from the third century AD using material from the previous century which seem to have direct relevance for a searcher after evidence for Roman instances of PTSD. Soldiering in the Roman Empire was more often than not a lifetime's profession and the law dealing with discharge from service is an obvious place to look for traces of these problems. Discharge from the Roman Army took three forms. The normal one was an honourable discharge (*missio honesta*) which came after 20–25 years' service. However, provision was also made for both dishonourable discharge (*missio ignominosa*) and, importantly here, discharge on medical grounds (*missio causaria*).[25]

Strikingly, *missio causaria* could be given for mental, as well as physical, reasons. The third-century jurist Ulpian defines the reason for such a discharge simply as *valetudo* or 'ill health'.[26] However, his near contemporary, Macer, expands on this, stating that such ill health was something that rendered its victim 'less fit', *minus idoneus*, for military service and was a product of a failure of either the mind or of the body—a *vitium animi vel corporis*—though sadly he does not define what should be regarded as such a *vitium*. The mid-third-century Emperor Gordian required that to obtain a *missio causaria*, a soldier had to submit to

[24] See K. van Lommel, 'The Recognition of Roman Soldiers' Mental Impairment', *Acta Classica* 56, 2013, 155–184. Many of the texts discussed here are conveniently gathered together in C.E. Brand, *Roman Military Law* (Austin and London: University of Texas Press, 1968).

[25] *Digest* (Macer) 49.16.13.3: Missionum generales causae sunt tres: honesta causaria ignominiosa. honesta est, quae tempore militiae impleto datur: causaria, cum quis vitio animi vel corporis minus idoneus militiae renuntiatur: ignominiosa causa est, cum quis propter delictum sacramento solvitur.

[26] *Digest* (Ulpian) 3.2.2.2: multa genera sunt missionum. est honesta, quae emeritis stipendiis vel ante ab imperatore indulgetur: est causaria, quae propter valetudinem laboribus militiae solvit.

an inspection by doctors, *medici*, whose conclusions were to be certified by a 'competent judge', *iudex competens*. The choice of language here suggests that the judge concerned was not a doctor, but probably a senior officer in the unit, perhaps the *praefectus castrorum* in the case of the legions, is intended. There was no return to service.[27] The inclusion of this condition may have been because such discharge was regarded as an easy passage to a veteran's privileges. Diocletian and Maximian were to restrict these to those who had served 20 years or more with the colours.[28]

Macer's notion of a *vitium corporis* is easy to understand. Incapacitating injuries sustained in battle would no doubt head the list of such problems.[29] Ulpian also includes deafness and dumbness which may well have been so inflicted or have been the product of disease.[30] A *vitium animi* however is much more difficult to define. The concept is found in Roman Law dealing with the sale of slaves where a variety of problems are discussed.[31] However the *vitia* listed there, for example, a disposition to religious fanaticism or thieving, are hardly grounds for an honourable discharge. Another example included is that of having suicidal tendencies which a slave merchant was compelled to reveal to his would-be clients. While such tendencies are an attested symptom of PTSD, as we shall see, attempted suicide in the Roman army generated only at best a dishonourable discharge, *missio ignominiosa*, and so this datum is of no help here. The obvious reason for a soldier's discharge on mental grounds is that of brain injury caused by head trauma. A Roman soldier's head, though well protected by his helmet, remained the most vulnerable part of his body, particularly given that slashing weapons were the weapons

27 *Codex Iustinianus,* 12.35.6: Imperator Gordianus Semel causaria missis militibus instauratio non solet concedi obtentu recuperatae valitudinis melioris, quando non temere dimittantur, nisi quos constet medicis denuntiantibus et iudice competente diligenter etiam investigante vitium contraxisse.

28 *Codex Iustinianus,* 7.64.9; 10.55.2–3.

29 Constantine exempted from the poll tax those who were invalided out of the service for this reason along with their wives, *AE* 1937 232 = *FIRA2* 94.

30 *Digest* 29.1.4.

31 See *Digest* 21.1, Cicero, *De Officiis* 3.17.

of choice for most of his opponents. While helmets are effective life-savers, they are much less effective in preventing concussion.[32] Roman head surgery was good for its time which suggests that battles would have produced a number of brain-damaged survivors and it is here above all that we should seek our unfortunate dischargees.[33] These sections of the *Digest* therefore, while interesting in that they show that the Roman army was aware of mental health problems, are of no help in isolating potential cases of PTSD.

However, returning to the question of suicide in the army, there is another series of legal texts of interest in the *Digest*. There is a considerable literature on suicide in the Roman world, but sadly, albeit understandably, it tends to concentrate on occasional suicides among the aristocracy. However, a reference in the *Digest* raises the question as to whether it was a problem within the lower ranks of the army. Suicide, sadly, is all too common among contemporary sufferers of PTSD and so its presence in discussions here raises the possibility that it could provide potential evidence for its existence in antiquity.

Section 6 of title 16 in book 49 of the *Digest* deals with crimes contrary to common military discipline (*disciplina communis*).[34] These are listed as: attacking a superior officer, wilful disobedience of an officer's commands, being the first to flee in battle, spying for the enemy, feigning sickness to avoid battle, wounding one's comrades, and failing to protect one's officers. Immediately after the discussion of wounding one's comrades, is the following subsection, translated here in full:

> Concerning one who has wounded himself or tried to kill himself in another way, the Emperor Hadrian has written that the circumstances must be clarified so that if he chose to die from inability to endure suffering (*impatientia doloris*), weariness of life (*taedium vitae*), disease (*morbus*), madness (*furor*), or shame (*pudor*) action should not be taken against him, but he should be discharged with ignominy. If nothing of the sort occurred, he should be executed. The death penalty should be remitted

[32] Je Yeong Sone et al., 'Helmet Efficacy Against Concussion and Traumatic Brain Injury: A Review', *Journal of Neurosurgery* 126.3, 2017, 661–1027.

[33] V.J. Belfiglio, 'Treatment of Traumatic Brain Injury in the Roman Army', *Balkan Military Medical Review* 18.4, 2015, 101–05.

[34] This section of the *Digest* is printed in full with an English translation in Brand, *Roman Military Law*.

> from those who have offended through wine or debauchery (*lascivia*) and they should be demoted.[35]

The last sentence has provoked some comment, but presumably refers to soldiers who have accidentally come close to killing themselves through drunkenness or horseplay: something poor for discipline, but hardly cases of attempted suicide at all, hence the less severe penalty exacted.

The logic of the section is clear—killing one's self would be to deprive the army of a soldier as much as wounding one's fellow-soldiers. As such, suicide was regarded as a form of desertion and hence attempted suicide was standardly seen as a capital offence. Hadrian's new provisions modified this approach by making exceptions to the general rule. It must be remembered that even these exceptions still retained the stigma attached to attempted suicide, as they resulted in a dishonourable discharge from the army not a *missio causaria*. Nevertheless, though a crime they remained, certain forms of suicide henceforth were no longer a capital crime. What is immediately noticeable is that arguably three out of the five categories where the emperor made exceptions—weariness of life, (*taedium vitae*), madness (*furor*), and shame (*pudor*)—are mental rather than physical problems, and all could correspond to symptoms commonly associated with PTSD. *Taedium vitae* is perhaps depression, *furor*, or irrational anger, is a common symptom of PTSD, as are feelings of guilt which could be subsumed under *pudor*.

The passage in the *Digest* is drawn from a lost work by the jurist Arrius Menander, *On Military Matters/De Re Militari* which was written at the beginning of the third century AD and regarded as a standard work on military law. It is also referred to by another third-century jurist Papinian:

> The deified Hadrian stated in a rescript that the will of a soldier who chose to die because he could no longer stand his pain or is weary of life is valid.[36]

[35] *Digest* 49.16.6.7: Qui se vulneravit vel alias mortem sibi conscivit, imperator Hadrianus rescripsit, ut modus eius rei statutus sit, ut, si impatientia doloris aut taedio vitae aut morbo aut furore aut pudore mori maluit, non animadvertatur in eum, sed ignominia mittatur, si nihil tale praetendat, capite puniatur. per vinum aut lasciviam lapsis capitalis poena remittenda est et militiae mutatio irroganda.

[36] Digest (Papinian) 29.1.34: Eius militis, qui doloris impatientia vel taedio vitae mori maluit, testamentum valere...divus Hadrianus rescripsit.

A further version of what should be the same ruling with a longer, but vaguer remit is found in the two jurists' near contemporary, Paulus:

> A soldier who turns his hand against himself, but with no success, unless he did this from inability to bear his suffering (*impatentia doloris*), disease (*morbus*), some other form of grief (*luctus*) or other cause (*alia causa*), shall be executed. Otherwise he is to be dismissed in ignomin.[37]

Here then is potential evidence for a long-standing and dangerous phenomenon within the Roman army. Certainly, one way of looking at these statements would be to see them as showing that attempted (and no doubt actual) suicide was a significant problem in the ranks. However, the context of these provisions needs to be considered. A further quotation from the Digest from Ulpian, again active in the third century, shows us the origins of this legislation, and it is a trail which takes us away from military instances of PTSD.

> For *constitutiones* make invalid the wills of those who have chosen to die rather than be condemned, on account of their consciousness of having committed a crime, although they die still citizens; but if someone [chooses to die] because they are tired of life (*taedium vitae*) or unable to bear ill-health (*valetudinis adversae impatientia*) or as a gesture (*iactatio*), like some philosophers, their situation is such that their wills are valid. And in a letter to Pomponius [Pompeius] Falco, the deified Hadrian laid down that this distinction applied to a soldier's will also.[38]

It is clear that Ulpian is once again referring to the same judgement of Hadrian as his fellow jurists have used. Given that suicide was regarded as a form of desertion in Roman military law, it abrogated the privilege of making a legally enforceable will granted to serving soldiers. As can be seen above, the suicide of criminals too made their wills invalid in the

[37] Digest (Paulus) 48.19.38.12: Miles, qui sibi manus intulit nec factum peregit, nisi impatientia doloris aut morbi luctusve alicuius vel alia causa fecerit, capite puniendus est: alias cum ignominia mittendus est.

[38] *Digest* 28.3.6.7: quod si quis taedio vitae vel valetudinis adversae impatientia vel iactationis, ut quidam philosophi, in ea causa sunt, ut testamenta eorum valeant. quam distinctionem in militis quoque testamento divus hadrianus dedit epistula ad pomponium falconem, ut, si quidem ob conscientiam delicti militaris mori maluit, irritum sit eius testamentum: quod si taedio vel dolore, valere testamentum aut, si intestato decessit, cognatis aut, si non sint, legioni ista sint vindicanda.

civilian world in normal circumstances. Hadrian, however, was eager that the law should reflect the context of actual events rather than simply be a set of rules which would be applied mechanically irrespective of circumstances and thus introduced changes to the law.[39] It was his *constitutio* which changed the law on suicide. The inclusion of suicide as a 'gesture' by 'certain philosophers' nods to the famous suicide of Socrates, but refers more directly to the society stoic philosopher, Euphrates, who was given permission to commit suicide by Hadrian as he was worn out by old age and ill health.[40] This is a classic case of *taedium vitae*, 'weariness of life', where the poor quality of life lived leaves an individual with the sense that life is no longer worth living. The philosopher then actively chooses death to assert his control over events and demonstrate his indifference to the material world.[41] It was a notion that appealed to Hadrian who said to himself to have attempted such a death at the end of his life.[42] From this passage of Ulpian, we can see that the emperor's rescript to Pomponius/Pompeius Falco[43] is a reply to a request for clarification, not the creation of extra legislation. Falco's wish was to know whether the new exemptions the emperor had made about suicide—note the use of a linking relative pronoun, '*quem distinctionem*'—also applied in the military sphere and the emperor answers in the affirmative.

Thus, we can see that Hadrian was not thinking about the army when he changed the law on suicide and that his rescript to Falco is simply putting into place a process of carrying over a set of civilian criteria into military law for the sake of legal tidiness. These tralatician elements include shame, *pudor*, and seemingly rage, *furor*, as we know that Hadrian

[39] See, for example, his decision to countenance manslaughter as opposed to murder, *Digest* 48.8.1.3.

[40] See Cassius Dio 69.8, Euphrates is praised by Pliny, *Epistulae*, 1.10, but harshly criticised by Philostratus, *Vitae Sophistorum* 1.7.

[41] See Seneca, *Epistulae Morales ad Lucilium,* 3.24, *ridiculum est currere ad mortem taedio vitae,* 'it is ridiculous to rush to death from a weariness of life'; *vir fortis ac sapiens non fugere debet e vita sed exire,* 'The brave and wise man ought not to flee from life but to leave it'.

[42] Scriptores Historiae Augustae, *Hadriani,* 24.

[43] 'Pomponius Falco' is probably to be identified with Quintus Roscius Murena Coelius Pompeius Falco. See *CIL* 10.6231 = *ILS* 1035.

granted that the will of a man who killed himself after killing his own son should be valid and such a case would encompass both these conditions.[44]

The derivative nature of the rescript therefore unfortunately gives us no firm evidence that any of its objects of concern was a frequent occurrence in the army. Nevertheless, there must have been a reason for Falco's inquiry in the first place. Given the reactive nature of Roman Law, it is likely that it was brought about as the result of a particular legal challenge. The best candidate is surely one brought by a potential financial beneficiary in the aftermath of a soldier's suicide due to an inability to bear pain, *impatentia doloris*. Roman military surgery was good for its times, but the lack of understanding of infection would have led to some horrendous instances of gangrene and the physical suffering concomitant to it. Disease too should never be underestimated as a killer of soldiers. In this period, it is likely to have accounted for more legionaries than the Germans and Parthians combined.[45] *Morbus* therefore is another distinct possibility for suicide.

While it is important to remember that Hadrian's categories ameliorating the shame of suicide are tralatician and so need not have any military bearing whatever, it is worth bearing in mind that all of them could occur in a military context without the presence of PTSD. Ridicule or disgust (including personal disgust) resulting from scars and wounds in a society where physical looks were often seen as a reflection of a man's personality could have generated enough *pudor*/shame to provoke suicide in some cases. As has been seen, Roman head surgery was relatively good and as such cases of *furor* (if they existed) are best explained as a product of surviving head trauma. Another possibility is that such acts were a response engendered by Roman cultural *mores* to perceived slights and insults to honour or as a way to recuperate one's honour. Such behaviour was noted by Emile Durkheim in his classic study on suicide and was most famously present in the Japanese practice of Seppuku. It is also, of course, to be found in the West embedded in the notion of 'doing the decent thing'.[46] Acting in this way may well be a result of military

[44] *Digest* 48.21.3.4.

[45] V.J. Belfiglio, 'Control of epidemics in the Roman army: 27 B.C.–A.D. 476', *International Journal of Community Medicine and Public Health* 4.5, 2017, 1387–91.

[46] E. Durkheim, E, *Le Suicide: étude de sociologie* (Paris: Alcan, 1897; reprinted, New York: The Free Press, 1951), p. 227; A. Rankin, *Seppuku: A History of Samurai Suicide* (Tokyo and New York: Kodansha International, 2011).

conditioning, but, even if that is the case, there is no link between such actions and PTSD. It is worth noting that, despite its discussion in ancient medical writers, *furor* is never linked there with military service.

The last of Hadrian's categories, *taedium vitae,* is perhaps the most difficult. This condition, as we have seen above, was normally brought on by physical failings of a sort which were less than extreme pain, but whose continual presence made life a burden. It is, in a way, easy to envisage cases like this in a military context. Wounds incurred in battle could lead to such a condition. One neglected possibility here is that of tinnitus.[47] The worst forms of tinnitus are often the product of head and neck trauma. Given what we have seen of Roman protection and surgery, such a condition is likely to have befallen some Roman troops. Understandably extreme tinnitus can lead to suicidal tendencies.

It must also be remembered that the Roman soldier was the most heavily loaded infantryman until those of the Great War. The yoke system used to carry his kit was not ergonomically efficient and carrying heavy weights in this way can significantly increase the number of spine injuries leading to chronic back pain.[48] Such a suicide provoked by such continuous low-level pain could be seen as a military version of Euphrates's death. This, indeed, could be seen as a sort of depression, but again it is not one engendered by PTSD. However, given that one could obtain a medical discharge from the army, such scenarios seem unlikely: it is more than likely that these conditions would produce a *missio causaria* rather than attempted suicide from *taedium vitae.*

We must therefore conclude that Roman legal texts while providing our best literary evidence into the world of the contemporary soldier, give no clear proof that PTSD was a significant problem in the Roman army. It would be foolish, of course, to assert that no Roman soldier was ever psychologically traumatised by his service, however it would be equally unwise to use material where there are other more obvious explanations

[47] P. Kreuzer, et al., 'Trauma-Associated Tinnitus', *Journal of Head Trauma Rehabilitation*, 29.5, 2014, 432–42.

[48] There is an extensive literature on this problem. See H.A. Orloff and C.M. Rapp, 'The Effects of Load Carriage on Spinal Curvature and Posture', *Spine* 29.12, 2004, 1325–29; R. Attwells, 'Influence of Carrying Heavy Loads on Soldier's Posture, Movements and Gait', *Ergonomics* 49, 2006, 1527–37; J.R. Meakin, et al., 'The Effect of Axial Load on the Sagittal Plane Curvature of the Upright Human Spine in Vivo', *Journal of Biomechanics* 41.13, 2008, 2850–54.

to hand as evidence to assert that this was a common problem in antiquity. The legal case for PTSD in the Roman army remains, like the existence of the syndrome itself, 'unproven' at best.

Bibliography

Attwells, R., et al., 'Influence of Carrying Heavy Loads on Soldier's Posture, Movements and Gait', *Ergonomics* 49, 2006, 1527–37.

Baughman Shively, S., et al., 'Characterisation of Interface Astroglial Scarring in the Human Brain After Blast Exposure: A Post-mortem Case Series', *The Lancet: Neurology* 15.9, 2016, 944–53.

Belfiglio, V. J., 'Treatment of Traumatic Brain Injury in the Roman Army', *Balkan Military Medical Review* 18.4, 2015, 101–05.

Belfiglio, V.J., 'Control of Epidemics in the Roman Army: 27 B.C.–A.D. 476', *International Journal of Community Medicine and Public Health* 4.5, 2017, 1387–91.

Bourne, P., *Men, Stress, and Vietnam* (Boston: Little, Brown, 1970).

Brand, C.E., *Roman Military Law* (Austin and London: University of Texas Press, 1968).

Denman A., *An Analysis of Roman Mutiny Narratives through Multiple Perspectives*, Unpublished MA thesis (MacMaster University, 2013).

Diouron, N., *Pseudo-César, Guerre d'Espagne* (Paris: Les Belles Lettres, 1999).

Durkheim, E, *Le Suicide: étude de sociologie* (Paris: Alcan, 1897; reprinted, New York: The Free Press, 1951).

Frazer, R.M., *The Trojan War: the Chronicles of Dictys of Crete and Dares the Phrygian* (Bloomington: Indiana University Press, 1966).

Fulkerson, L., *No Regrets: Remorse in Classical Antiquity* (Oxford: Oxford University Pressm 2013).

Goldsworthy, A.K., *The Roman Army at War, 100 BC-AD 200* (Oxford: Oxford University Press, 1996).

Koon, S., *Infantry Combat in Livy's Battle Narratives (British Archaeological Reports, International Series 2071)* (Oxford: BAR Publishing, 2010).

Kreuzer, P., et al., 'Trauma-Associated Tinnitus', *Journal of Head Trauma Rehabilitation*, 29.5, 2014, 432–42.

Holmes, R., *Acts of War: The Behaviour of Men in Battle* (London: Cassell, 2003).

Howell, A., 'The Demise of PTSD: From Governing through Trauma to Governing Resilience', *Alternatives* 37.3, 2012, 214–26.

Lazarus, R. S. and Folkman, S., *Stress, Appraisal, and Coping* (New York: Springer, 1984).

Lord Southborough, *Report of the War Office Committee of Enquiry into 'Shell Shock'* (London: HMSO 1922, reprinted 2014).

Meakin, J.R., et al., 'The Effect of Axial Load on the Sagittal Plane Curvature of the Upright Human Spine in Vivo', *Journal of Biomechanics* 41.13, 2008, 2850–54.

Mommsen, T., *The Provinces of the Roman Empire: From Caesar to Diocletian,* volume1, (London: MacMillan & Co., 1909).

Mora-Lebrun, F., 'Joseph of Exeter: Troy through Dictys and Dares', in Simms, R.C. (ed), *Brill's Companion to Prequels, Sequels, and Retellings of Classical Epic* (Leiden: Brill, 2018), pp. 115–33.

Orloff, H.A. and Rapp, C.M., 'The Effects of Load Carriage on Spinal Curvature and Posture', *Spine* 29.12, 2004, 1325–29.

Peacock, E.J. and Wong, P.T.P., 'Anticipatory Stress: The Relation of Locus of Control, Optimism, and Control Appraisals to Coping', *Journal of Research in Personality* 30, 1996, 204–22.

Prosperi, V., 'The Place of the Father: the Reception of Homer in the Renaissance Canon', in E. Morra (ed), *Building the Canon though the Classics* (Leiden: Brill, 1988), 47–69.

Rankin, A., *Seppuku: A History of Samurai Suicide* (Tokyo and New York: Kodansha International, 2011).

Rice Holmes, T., *The Roman Republic and the Founder of the Empire*, vol. 2 (Oxford: Clarendon Press, 1923).

Rotter, J. B., *Social Learning and Clinical Psychology* (Englewood Cliffs, NJ: Prentice-Hall, 1954).

Shay, J., *Achilles in Vietnam* (New York: Maxwell Macmillan International, 1994).

Sherman, N., *Stoic Warriors* (Oxford: Oxford University Press, 2005)

Sone, Je Yeong, et al., 'Helmet Efficacy Against Concussion and Traumatic Brain Injury: A Review', *Journal of Neurosurgery* 126.3, 2017, 661–1027.

Storch, R.H., 'The Author of the 'De Bello Hispaniensi': A Cavalry Officer?', *Acta Classica* 20, 1977, 201–04.

Stouffer S.A., et al., *The American Soldier: Combat and Its Aftermath* (New York: Wiley, 1949).

Van Hoof, 'The Caesar of the 'Bellum Hispaniense'', *Mnemosyne,* 27.2, 1974, 123–38.

van Lommel, K., 'Heroes and Outcasts: Ambiguous Attitudes Towards Impaired and Disfigured Roman Veterans', *Classical World* 109.1, 2015, 91–117.

van Lommel, K., 'The Recognition of Roman Soldiers' Mental Impairment', *Acta Classica* 56, 2013, 155–84.

Terrible but Unavoidable? Combat Trauma and a Change to Legal Proscriptions on Roman Military Suicide Under Hadrian

Joanne E. Ball

One of the lesser-discussed aspects of Roman military life is the phenomenon of suicide among enlisted soldiers, in service but off the battlefield. The subject is little discussed in antiquity. On the rare occasions where military suicide is mentioned, it is usually in the context of soldiers who killed themselves during (or shortly after) a devastating Roman defeat in battle, or when surrounded by the enemy without hope of rescue. Little is said, or known, of soldiers who committed suicide off the battlefield when they were not at immediate threat of shame or death—and although not discussed in any detail in the historical record, it is clear that such actions did happen, and that it became an issue that the Roman legal system eventually found it necessary to address by the first decades of the second century AD.

The military reforms of Augustus created a standing army for the Roman Empire, which led to new challenges with regard to the treatment of soldiers over the course of not just a single war, but over several decades

J. E. Ball (✉)
University of Liverpool, Liverpool, UK
e-mail: j.e.ball@liverpool.ac.uk

O. Rees et al. (eds.), *Combat Stress in Pre-modern Europe*, Mental Health in Historical Perspective,
https://doi.org/10.1007/978-3-031-09947-2_6

of service in the army. The longer-term physical and mental well-being of soldiers became an issue for the Roman military institution in a way it had not been during the Republican period, where men were recruited for individual periods of conflict and then discharged back into civilian life. The psychological impact of warfare would have become much more likely than before to affect soldiers still under active service, including military suicide. From the late first century BC to the early second century AD, all Roman soldiers who committed suicide off the battlefield, whatever their reason for doing so, were considered to have deserted the army, and suffered post-mortem legal censure as a result. Their wills were declared invalid,[1] and their property therefore automatically forfeit to the state instead of any family or other beneficiaries originally named in the document.[2]

This situation changed during the reign of Hadrian (AD 117–138), due to a legal rescript introduced by the emperor, which allowed the wills of Roman soldiers to remain valid if their suicide was prompted by severe physical pain, or 'tiring of life'. Why Hadrian introduced this ruling is unknown, but the nature of the rescript makes it clear that it was a response to real cases happening in the military community, rather than an abstract ruling put forward as a solution to a hypothetical future issue. The rescript served to divide Roman military suicides into two categories: those which were 'sanctioned' by the state, in as much as the will of the soldier was allowed to stand, and those which were not, in which case the will would be rendered invalid, and the soldier's beneficiaries denied any testaments made to them. The outcome would be decided based on the cause of the suicide. As the rescript notes, it was not just in cases of physical pain that suicides were treated this way, but also in cases where the psychological health of soldiers was an issue. It is the aim of this paper to explore Hadrian's rescript in greater detail, suggesting that it represents a Roman recognition of some level of combat trauma among soldiers in

[1] K. Van Lommel, 'The Recognition of Roman Soldiers' Mental Impairment', *Acta Classica* 56, 2013, 161.

[2] Given that military marriage was officially still banned during Hadrian's reign (under a rule passed under Augustus which would not be rescinded until the reign of Caracalla in the early third century AD), the beneficiaries of serving soldiers should not have included wives and children, although in reality soldiers seem to have started families anyway, who presumably they would make provision for in their wills (on military marriage see S.E. Phang, *The Marriage of Roman Soldiers (13 B.C.–A.D. 235): Law and Family in the Imperial Army* (Leiden: Brill, 2001).

the Roman army—significant enough in itself—but also that this trauma could be a direct cause of military suicide off the battlefield, perhaps long after the battle had been fought.

Roman Military Mental Health

Substantial academic attention has been devoted in recent years to the psychology and mental health of the average Roman soldier, including the experience of battle,[3] generalised combat trauma,[4] and whether they suffered from PTSD during or after their military service.[5] Much of the research assumes that there should be some degree of universality in military experience between that of the Roman world and better-documented later warfare, meaning that broad parallels, at least, can be drawn, although there is scholarly debate about how far this process can be pushed, particularly given the disparities between the ancient evidence and its more modern counterpart.[6]

[3] P. Sabin, 'The Face of Roman Battle', *The Journal of Roman Studies* 90, 2000, 1–17; Daly 2002; S.M. Heidenreich and J.P. Roth 'The Neurophysiology of Panic on the Ancient Battlefield', in L.L. Brice (ed), *New Approaches to Greek and Roman Warfare* (Hoboken, NJ: Wiley-Blackwell, 2020), pp. 127–38.

[4] A.D. Lee, 'Morale and the Roman Experience of Battle', in A.B. Lloyd (ed), *Battle in Antiquity* (Swansea: Classical Press of Wales), pp. 199–217. S. Chrissanthos, 'Aeneas in Iraq: Comparing the Roman and Modern Battle Experience', in M.B., Cosmopoulos (ed), *Experiencing War: Trauma and Society from Ancient Greece to the Iraq War* (Chicago: Ares, 2007), pp. 225–57.

[5] A. Melchior, 'Caesar in Vietnam: Did Roman Soldiers Suffer from Post-traumatic Stress Disorder?', *Greece & Rome* 58.2, 2011, 209–23; L.A. Tritle, '"Ravished Minds" in the Ancient World', in P. Meineck and D. Konstan (eds), *Combat Trauma and the Ancient Greeks* (New York: Palgrave, 2014), pp. 87–103; V.J. Belfiglio, 'Post traumatic Stress Disorder and Acute Stress Disorder in Army: Lessons for Modern Armies'. *Balkan Military Medical Review* 18.3, 2015, 65–71. Diagnosing PTSD in the Roman world is difficult because little is documented of soldier's lives after they left the army; most attempts to do so are based on extrapolation from a limited range of sources, analysing their (likely) experiences while enlisted, and creating parallels with more modern (and better documented) warfare (e.g. L.A. Tritle, 'Soldiers' Home: Life After Battle', in L.L. Brice (ed), *New Approaches to Greek and Roman Warfare* (Hoboken, NJ: Wiley-Blackwell, 2020), pp. 53–64; Melchior, 'Caesar in Vietnam', 211–12).

[6] Example 'Even though ancient and modern soldiers are separated by great gulfs in time, culture, and technology, warfare had a dramatic effect on those in combat and, despite the above differences, human beings generally respond in similar ways to what in many respects were similar military experiences' Chrissanthos, 'Aeneas in Iraq', p. 225; Heidenreich and Roth, 'Neurophysiology of Panic', note the neurobiological similarities

Although there is debate on how best to understand the psychological impact of military life on the average Roman soldier, there are hints in the ancient sources that battlefield experiences could have longer-term impacts on mental health. While the potential for Roman soldiers to feel fear before and during battle has been recognised,[7] the impact of this emotion away from the battlefield has been little considered. Previous scholarship has suggested that many Roman soldiers were psychologically 'toughened' against combat-related trauma by their exposure pre-enlistment to injury and death.[8] The close bonds within the military community, particularly within the *contubernium*, would have provided support for soldiers affected by trauma.[9] Nevertheless, elements of Roman military life did have the potential to prove traumatic.

There does seem to have been a general awareness in the Roman world that military life could have a negative psychological impact on soldiers, although the causes are not discussed by either historical or legal sources.[10] By the first century AD, psychological injury, like its physical counterpart, had been formally recognised as a valid reason for a soldier being honourably discharged from the army on medical grounds (*missio causaria*), before completing his full term of service; until the third century AD this counted as an honourable discharge with full benefits no matter how long the soldier had served.[11] The military community no doubt gave Roman soldiers some resilience to the trauma of military

between ancient and modern soldiers. Although see J. Crowley, 'Beyond the Universal Soldier: Combat Trauma in Classical Antiquity', in P. Meineck and D. Konstan (eds), *Combat Trauma and the Ancient Greeks* (New York: Palgrave, 2014), pp. 105–30 for the argument that the cultural background of ancient soldiers may have impacted their responses to conflict. A similar debate on PTSD and combat trauma is currently underway in the context of ancient Greek warfare—see O. Rees, 'We Need to Talk About Epizelus: 'PTSD' and the Ancient World', *Medical Humanities* 46, 2020, 46–54.

[7] J.C.N. Coulston, 'Courage and Cowardice in the Roman Imperial Army', *War in History* 20.1, 2013, 7–31.

[8] Melchior, 'Caesar in Vietnam', 222–223.

[9] On the *contubernium* see A. Goldsworthy, *The Roman Army at War, 100 BC–AD 200* (Oxford: Clarendon, 1996), pp. 252–54.

[10] K. Van Lommel, 'The Recognition of Roman Soldiers' Mental Impairment', *Acta Classica* 56, 2013, 155–84.

[11] K. Van Lommel, 'The Terminology of the Medical Discharge and an Identity Shift among the Roman Disabled Veterans', *Ancient History Bulletin* 27, 2013, 65–74. The provision seems to have been introduced in either the Late Republican or Early Imperial periods—certainly by AD 70, when it is references on a military diploma, and likely as

life, potentially mitigating the psychological impact of their experiences on the battlefield—but was this enough to overcome all forms of combat trauma? The historical evidence would suggest not.

Suicide in the Roman Army

In absolute terms, the suicide of soldiers was not a moral problem for the Roman army. Suicide was, in some cases, socially acceptable in the Roman world, with a wide range of reasons cited in the ancient sources, including physical and mental pain, shame, frenzy, loyalty, old age (tiring of life), and loyalty to a (defeated) leader or cause.[12] In other cases, where suicide could be linked to a guilty conscience or a perceived general weakness, it was received more negatively (if still not considered an immoral act, as such). In these cases, the deceased might not receive the same burial rites as the other military dead and were not supposed to be mourned; they would be counted among the 'discontented dead'.[13] It was not the act itself that invited censure, but the reasoning behind it which formed the dividing line between socially acceptable suicide and its distained counterpart.

There were some situations in which it was considered acceptable, even preferable, for a Roman soldier to commit suicide. As previously mentioned, these were usually situations associated with overwhelming defeat on the battlefield, particularly when captivity, torture, and/or enslavement by the enemy was likely. It has been claimed that Roman soldiers—both rank-and-file and officers—would be likely to kill themselves after an overwhelming defeat on the battlefield, to avoid both the shame of defeat and captivity,[14] although it has recently been argued that

part of the military reforms under Augustus: Ibid., 73. Under Caracalla, a requirement of 20+ years of service was required for full retirement benefits.

[12] A.J.L. Van Hooff, *From Autothanasia to Suicide: Self-Killing in Classical Antiquity* (London: Routledge, 1990), pp. 79–132.

[13] V.M. Hope, *Roman Death: The Dying and the Dead in Ancient Rome* (London: Continuum, 2009), pp. 57–60.

[14] van Hooff *From Autothanasia*, 87–89, 109–110; Hill 2004, 198; Goldsworthy, *Roman Army*, 262–263; Coulston, 'Courage and Cowardice'; van Lommel, 'Recognition', 160–161. The 'conquer or die' approach is reflected in the tendency from the Late Republic onward to refuse state ransom of captured soldiers, as documented by Cicero (*De Officiis*, 3.114). Captured Roman soldiers would also lose their citizenship and associated rights while in enemy hands, including the validity of their wills (Ulpian

this reason for military suicide has been vastly over-estimated.[15] Most of the historical incidents of Roman military suicide take place in the context of comprehensive battlefield defeat, where soldiers were left with little choice between death at their own hands, or those of the enemy. At the Battle of Trasimene (217 BC), soldiers still alive in the late stages of the battle eventually asked their comrades to kill them, preferring this to capture or slaughter at the hands of the Carthaginians.[16] In 54 BC, during the Ambioric Revolt, the Legio V was surrounded in camp by the Eburones and opted to commit mass suicide rather than fall into the hands of the enemy—according to Caesar, they literally 'despaired of safety'.[17] After defeat in an ambush at the Teutoburg Forest (Germany) in AD 9, many of the soldiers from the three legions caught in the attack committed suicide, both by their own hands and by letting the enemy cut them down without resistance.[18] Shortly after, Caldus Caelius, a Roman soldier captured by the Germans, is said to have killed himself by bringing a section of his chains down on his head so hard that he fell down dead.[19] These cases share in common the fact that in each the Roman soldiers who committed suicide were faced with overwhelming defeat, in which death may have seemed a preferable alternative to the fate they would face if captured by the enemy.[20] As such, these suicides can be seen not as a last-resort, but rational, responses to the military reality, *contra* to

Digest 49.15.19.2), unless they were captured by bandits or pirates: B.D. Shaw, 'Bandits in the Roman Empire', in R. Osborne (ed), *Studies in Ancient Greek and Roman Society* (Cambridge: Cambridge University Press, 2004), pp. 342–43.

[15] S.H. Rauh, 'The Tradition of Suicide in Rome's Foreign Wars', *TAPA* 145, 2015, 383–410. Rauh argues that military suicide was not typical after general defeats (outside of civil war), only in overwhelming situations on the battlefield—and that soldiers were motivated by the desire to avoid pain, rather than shame.

[16] Polybius, 3.84.10.

[17] Caesar, *Bellum Gallicum*, 5.37.6 '*Desperata salus*'—sometimes translated as 'despairing of deliverance'.

[18] Cassius Dio, 56.22.1.

[19] Velleius Paterculus, 2.120.6.

[20] Given the descriptions of the tortures visited on Roman soldiers captured after the Battle of the Teutoburg (Tacitus, *Annales*, 1.61; Florus *Epitome* 2.30.37) it is unsurprising that individuals would want to avoid captivity where possible, even if the literary descriptions do not reflect reality, only the perception of 'barbarian' treatment of prisoners.

previous interpretations which saw these suicides as a panicked or traumatised reaction,[21] or a fear of shame in defeat.[22] In any case, these suicides do not seem to have drawn any societal censure—indeed, in most cases the soldiers are praised for having the courage to die under their own terms.

But away from the battlefield, soldiers in the Roman army were not permitted the same freedoms with regards to suicide as their civilian counterparts—at least, not without legal penalties for themselves or their families. This seems a consequence of the Roman soldier's individual relationship to the state—or rather, the fact that, while enlisted, a soldier was the property of the state, and suicide was therefore an act of treason against the state.[23] Soldiers who attempted suicide but survived could face censure and even—counterintuitively—execution, although in many cases, if they were thought to have a valid excuse for their attempt, they would instead receive a dishonourable discharge from the army, with none of the benefits they might otherwise have expected to receive after service.[24] Up until the early second century AD, soldiers who successfully committed suicide would have their wills declared invalid, confiscating any financial benefits that would have fallen to their beneficiaries and giving them instead to the state—but under Hadrian this changed, to allow a small number of circumstances under which soldier's wills did not automatically become invalid after their suicide.

Hadrian's Rescript—*Digest* 28.3.6.7 and 29.1.34

The Hadrianic rescript on military suicide is preserved in the Justinian *Digest* (or *Pandects*), a collection of legal writings compiled in the AD 530 s at the order of the Byzantine emperor Justinian I as part of an ambitious project to codify Roman law and standardise its use.[25] The rescript is mentioned twice in the *Digest*, both times in sections discussing

[21] Heidenreich and Roth, 'Neurophysiology of Panic', 136.

[22] Rauh, 'The Tradition', 404–08.

[23] Van Lommel, 'Recognition', 160.

[24] Van Hooff, *From Autothansia*, 84.

[25] W. Kaiser, 'Justinian and the *Corpus Iuris Civilis*', in D. Johnston (ed), *The Cambridge Companion to Roman Law* (Cambridge: Cambridge University Press, 2015), 119–48.

the validity of wills in general, and military wills more specifically. At the time Hadrian ordered the rescript, military wills would still have been a relatively new phenomenon in the Roman world. Soldiers had only been legally permitted to make wills from the reign of Titus (AD79–81), aside from a temporary period under Julius Caesar, and the practice was still sufficiently recent that each subsequent emperor had felt it necessary to reconfirm its continuation.[26] The making of military wills was subject to complex guidelines about when they were and were not valid, which are discussed in detail in the *Digest*.[27]

The rescript discussed in this paper was made at an unknown point in the reign of Hadrian. It legally sanctioned the suicide of Roman soldiers under a certain, limited range of circumstances, by allowing their will and testaments to remain valid after their death, *contra* to previous practice. On this provision, Ulpian documented:

> And in a letter to Pomponius [Pompeius] Falco, the deified Hadrian laid down that this distinction applied to a soldier's will also, so that if he chose to die on account of his consciousness of having committed a military crime, his will should be ineffectual; but if it was **because he was tired of life or because of pain** [*quod si taedio vel dolore*], his will is valid, or if he died intestate, his [belongings] are to be claimed for his cognates, or if there are none, for his legion.[28]

The rescript was confirmed by an extract from another jurist, Papinian, in a further section of the *Digest*:

> The deified Hadrian stated in a rescript that the will of a soldier who has preferred to die, **because he can no longer stand his pain or is weary of life** [*qui doloris impatientia vel taedio vitae*], is valid, or if he has died intestate, his property is claimed by those who are called to the succession by statute.[29]

[26] *Digest* 29.1.1.

[27] *Digest* 29.1.1–44.

[28] *Digest* 28.3.6.7; A. Watson (ed, trans), *The Digest of Justinian*. 4 volumes (Philadelphia: University of Philadelphia Press, 1998) of T. Mommsen, *The Digest of Justinian Latin Text* (Philadelphia: University of Philadelphia Press, 1985); my emphasis.

[29] *Digest* 29.1.34; trans. Watson, *Digest* (1998) of Mommsen, *Digest* (1985); my emphasis.

Unfortunately, the legal codes do not preserve what were considered to be acceptable reasons for military suicide—this is fairly characteristic of these sources, which record the letter of the law, not the motivations behind it. How the rescript was policed is equally unclear, and little detail is given about the process for deciding whether the legal criteria for sanctioned suicide had been satisfied, including who would have made the decision, or what evidence they might consult. Van speculates that fellow soldiers could be consulted about the mental state of the deceased, particularly the other members of his *contubernium*, but this is extrapolated from the strength of bonds within this group rather than a reflection of specific evidence.[30] However it was policed, the rescript under Hadrian essentially recognised extenuating circumstances by which a military suicide should not be received with further punishment visited on the soldier's beneficiaries—but why was this legal change considered desirable or necessary?

'Tiring of (Military) Life'

Hadrian's rescript gives two circumstances under which Roman soldiers could commit suicide off the battlefield and still maintain the validity of their will: because of '(physical) pain' (*dolore/inpatientia doloris*), and through being 'tired/weary of life' (*taedium vitae*)—while specifying that it did not cover soldiers who killed themselves in anticipation of punishment for a military crime. These were among the categories recognised as understandable reasons for civilian suicide, but had not previously been acknowledged in a military context, with soldiers who committed suicide for these reasons posthumously punished by having their wills rescinded. Under Hadrian, the situation changed, with a certain leeway on suicide extended to soldiers who committed suicide under what might be considered 'mitigating circumstances'. The wording of the rescript suggests that no distinction was made between citizen legionary soldiers and non-citizen auxiliaries, nor that there were any preconditions over, for example, length of service prior to suicide, or proof of exposure to a particular scenario, although it is possible that in reality there were some associated conditions which have not been preserved in the legal text.

[30] Van Lommel, 'Recognition', 162.

The inclusion of the rescript in the Digest shows that these allowances were not theoretical, but reflect jurist's rulings drawn from actual cases, meaning that the rescript was introduced to deal with the real-life phenomenon of Roman military suicide.[31] However, allowances were not extended to all suicides, only those which satisfied a predetermined criteria laid out by Hadrian—suggesting that not all incidents occurred for these reasons. Certainly, this rescript should not be seen as a state-sanction of suicide committed for any reason, particularly to avoid punishment for some other nefarious action, which remained particularly frowned-upon. It is clear that the rescript was not intended to only cover suicides resulting from physical pain, but also those deriving from mental health or psychological issues—otherwise, there would be no need to include this as a distinctive category. Given the brutal nature of Roman warfare, it is easy to see how soldiers could have sustained physical injuries that would have resulted in severe chronic pain, but which did not qualify them for discharge on medical grounds.[32] However, it was not only physical pain that was covered, but also psychological conditions, broadly described as 'tired of life'—which seems to be a recognition of mental health issues that could, and did, drive soldiers to suicide.

Being 'tired of life' as a reason for suicide in a Roman civilian context is usually the result of old age, with various ailments that made life physically and mentally unbearable; in the written sources, it is an affliction often discussed—and suffered—by philosophers.[33] However, in the military context, we are likely looking at a different phenomenon. The age profile of Roman soldiers suggests that this is not a case of old-age stripping the meaning from life, leading to a generalised desire to die. Recruits to the Roman army were typically in their late teens or early twenties on enlistment, meaning that most of those who survived their full term of service would have been retired from the military by their 50th

[31] Ibid., 162.

[32] For the impact of Roman weapons on the human body see S.T. James, 'The Point of the Sword: What Roman-Era Weapons Could Do to Bodies—And Why They Often Didn't', in A.W. Busch and H.J. Schalles (eds), *Waffen in Aktion. Akten der 16. Internationalen Roman Military Equipment Conference (ROMEC). Xantener Berichte* 16, 2010, 41–54.

[33] Although the conditions in themselves were typically not (immediately) terminal. See van Hooff, *From Autothanasia*, pp. 121–23.

birthday.[34] Even if we accept that military life could have made soldiers old before their time, it is far from certain that by this age soldiers would have reached the point at which mind and body began to fall apart—and if so, the field operation and effectiveness of the Roman army would need to be seriously reconsidered. There is nothing in the wider historical record to suggest that most Roman soldiers remained enlisted past the point of age-related infirmity in the second century AD. So, if 'tiring of life' seems unlikely to reflect old age in the Roman army, what else could the clause be describing?

As we can suggest with a high degree of probability that the phrase refers to a psychological rather than physical condition, an alternative explanation is that 'tiring of life' is related to the mental health of soldiers, in response to their experiences during military service, including longer-term combat trauma. It would not necessarily have been the result of a single stressor event, or a reflection of independent mental health issues, but rather, the result of a slow cumulation of trauma during a series of (potentially individually unremarkable) events.[35] Certainly, Roman soldiers were exposed to situations in conflict, both on and off the battlefield, from which—to modern perceptions, at least—a degree of psychological trauma seems almost inevitable, no matter how hardened a soldier was by experiences from both his early and military lives. But is there sufficient evidence to suggest that Roman soldiers were affected by significant levels of combat trauma—and that these would have been sufficient to lead them to suicide?

[34] W. Scheidel, 'Marriage, Families, and Survival: Demographic Aspects', in P. Erdkamp (ed), *A Companion to the Roman Army* (Oxford: Blackwell, 2007), pp. 417–34. Although we have isolated incidents of older soldiers in the Roman army (either because they had been recruited later in life, or had overstayed beyond the normal term of service), this does not appear to have been common practice, despite complaints in some sources (e.g. Tac. *Ann.* 1.34) that soldiers were being kept in the army into their old age. T.G. Parkin, *Old Age in the Roman World: A Cultural and Social History* (Baltimore: Johns Hopkins University Press, 2003) notes that there was no universally agreed number at which 'old age' began; K. Cokayne, *Experiencing Old Age in Ancient Rome* (London: Routledge, 2003), pp. 11–33 suggests that it was judged on appearance and feeling rather than a biological age.

[35] A historical survey of 'tiredness of life' found that in most contexts the concept was used to describe suicide resulting from psychological rather than physical pain, often over an extended period of time: S. Pridmore, T.T. Money and W. Pridmore, 'Tedium Vitae [L: tired of life] Suicide', *Dynamics of Human Health* 4, 2017. https://journalofhealth.co.nz/wp-content/uploads/2017/09/DHH_Tedium-vitae_Saxby.pdf. Date accessed 22 December 2021.

Roman Combat Trauma

A third century AD funerary epigram from Cohors Breucorum (modern Tagremaret, Algeria) dedicated to a soldier named Ulpius Optatus provides a moving example of the impact of combat trauma in the ancient world.[36] Written in irregular verse, it briefly documents the military career of Optatus, before documenting his death, in battle, in what sounds like a suicide mission: 'As he unleashed his excessive anger in its entirety, that familiar rage of battle itself sent this young Roman straight into enemy-inflicted wounds'.[37] The final part of the inscription is damaged, leaving the end of the story slightly unclear, but of the traces that survive, Optatus appears to have died as a result of this attack—and the battle-frenzy which drove him towards the enemy with seemingly little regard for his own survival. The episode reads as an almost classic example of a soldier driven by trauma to excessive anger in battle, as a result of psychological traumas already sustained as a result of his military service.

Although there are justifiable concerns about applying modern psychological diagnoses to ancient (military) societies it is clear that combat trauma was experienced by at least some Roman soldiers.[38] Recognition of this fact does not rely purely on (potentially problematic) retrospective diagnoses of psychological conditions, because the evidence is clear that elements of combat trauma were recognised in the Roman world. As the Hadrianic rescript demonstrates, both the military and legal systems came to recognise and accept that some soldiers were driven to suicide as a result of their experiences in the army—for their 'tiring of life to become so overwhelming that they could no longer continue living. Although it is impossible to say with complete certainty what exact psychological trauma Roman soldiers were exposed to in their military lives, we can—with caution—explore some of the scenarios that may have triggered episodes of trauma, particularly those which may have had a longer-term impact on their mental health.

It would be easy to attribute psychological trauma among the Roman military to their experiences in battle. Roman warfare could be brutal,

[36] *CIL* VIII 21,562 = *CLE* 520; thanks are due to Peter Kruschwitz, who discussed this inscription in his blog *The Petrified Muse*.

[37] 'cum suam totam nimium / depend[ere]t iram obvius ipse furo[r] / pugnae Romanum iuvenem per / hostica vulnera misit'.

[38] Crowley, 'Beyond the Universal Soldier'.

and involved high levels of violence against both combatants and civilians.[39] There would be no shortage of potential trauma for almost any soldier caught up in active combat—battle in the Roman world must have been a terrifying experience, even for experienced soldiers, from the noise, smells, sounds, to the ever-present risk of pain and death. Psychological combat trauma may not have resulted from a single, devastating episode, but could accumulate over several, even many, engagements. The exact experience of the average Roman soldier in battle is difficult to reconstruct with any accuracy, as there are no written accounts from this perspective which survive; at best, we can infer from the wider historical narratives about the 'soldier's eye view' of battle. It would have been loud and disorientating, with soldiers vulnerable to injury and death from missiles—from threats they could not even see—as well as in hand-to-hand fighting[40]; many of the wounds that could be received in battle would be exceedingly painful.[41] It has been suggested that the majority of soldiers would have been more preoccupied with staying alive than actually fighting, consistent with studies from wars in much later history.[42] The historical record shows that under certain circumstances the Roman army was vulnerable to panic on the battlefield,[43] and a significant amount of the substantial training soldiers received aimed to reduce both the probability and impact of panic during combat.[44] The creation of strong community bonds within the military, particularly among the *contuburnium*, was no doubt intended to further increase the resilience of Roman soldiers in battle; how far these measures continued to support the mental health of soldiers outside combat is unknown.

[39] On brutality in Roman warfare see G. Baker, G., *Spare No One: Mass Violence in Roman Warfare* XX (Lanham: Rowman & Littlefield, 2020); for the Roman experience of battle, see Goldsworthy, *Roman Army*, esp. pp. 170–282; Lee, 'Morale'; Sabin, 'The Face of Roman Battle'.

[40] Sabin, 'The Face of Roman Battle'; Chrissanthos, 'Aeneas in Iraq', pp. 231–35.

[41] On the anthropological impact of ancient battle on the human body, albeit in a Greek context, see M.A. Liston, 'Skeletal Evidence for the Impact of Battle on Soldiers and Non-Combatants', in L.L. Brice (ed), *New Approaches to Greek and Roman Warfare* (Hoboken, NJ.: Wiley-Blackwell, 2020), pp. 81–94.

[42] Goldsworthy, *Roman Army*, pp. 219–22.

[43] Heidenreich and Roth, 'Neurophysiology of Panic', 136.

[44] S.E. Phang, *Roman Military Service: Ideologies of Discipline in the Late Republic and Early Principate* (Cambridge: Cambridge University Press, 2008).

There is little evidence from antiquity to suggest that soldiers were traumatised by the act of killing the enemy in battle, although it should be noted that the natures of the historical sources which have survived from antiquity give relatively little scope for this area of enquiry. It has been argued that in the ancient Greek context soldiers were psychologically protected against issues with killing the enemy by the societal norms and conditioning which they had grown up with.[45] Over the course of the Imperial period, as Roman soldiers became predominantly recruited from the provinces, substantial effort was made to 'dehumanise' the non-Roman enemy in art, language, and literature—such as, for example, the 'barbarians' being ridden over on cavalrymen tombstones,[46] captives portrayed on legionary distance markers[47] from the Antonine Wall,[48] and scenes of torture, execution, and dismemberment on the Columns of Trajan and Marcus Aurelius in Rome.[49] These artistic motifs may have served to provide a necessary buffer between the Roman soldier and the enemies he killed—particularly as, over the course of the first few centuries AD, recruits were increasingly drawn from the populations that they would later face in battle.[50]

The nature of Roman warfare also evolved over the course of the early Imperial period, leading up to the changes under Hadrian. From the late

[45] Crowley, 'Beyond the Universal Soldier'.

[46] I. Ferris, 'Insignificant Others: Images of Barbarians on Military Art from Roman Britain', in K. Meadows, C. Lemke and J. Heron (eds), *TRAC 96: Proceedings of the Sixth Annual Theoretical Roman Archaeology Conference* (Oxford: Oxbow Books, 1997), pp. 22–28.

[47] Stones inscribed with text recording building work carried out on the frontier by men from the legions, often decorated with relief sculpture depicting military scenes.

[48] D.J. Breeze and I. Ferris, 'They Think it's All Over. The Face of Victory on the British Frontier', *Journal of Conflict Archaeology* 11.1, 2016, 19–39; L. Campbell, 'Reading the Writing on the Wall: Discovering New Dimensions to the Antonine Wall Distance Sculptures', *Journal of Ancient History and Archaeology* 7, 2020, 46–75.

[49] I. Ferris, 'Suffering in Silence: The Political Aesthetics of Pain in Antonine Art'. *Journal of Conflict Archaeology* 1, 2005, 67–92. It is worth remembering that most—or all—of these monuments would also have been colourised in antiquity, adding to their visual effect—see L. Campbell, 'Polychromy on the Antonine Wall Distance sculptures: non-destructive Identification of pigments on Roman reliefs', *Britannia* 51, 2020, 175–201.

[50] For Roman auxiliary recruitment and service see I.P. Haynes, *Blood of the Provinces: The Roman Auxilia and the Making of Provincial Society from Augustus to the Severans* (Oxford: Oxford University Press, 2013).

Republican period onward, Rome's increasing activity in the provinces resulted in the predominant form of warfare evolving from conventional to asymmetric, against indigenous forces who were often numerically superior, but technologically and organisationally inferior. This exposed the Roman army to more frequent irregular engagements, particularly ambushes, which may have taken an even greater psychological toll on individual soldiers than pitched battle would have done. When they were not at war, soldiers would still have been required to conduct patrols, during which they would have been vulnerable to attack. During periods of conflict and unrest, soldiers may not even have been safe in their forts—one military tombstone from Ambleside (Britain) commemorates a soldier who was killed 'in the fort by the enemy', probably during an attack on the installation in an uprising at some point in the second or third century AD.[51] These low-level but constant stresses may have had a significant impact on individual soldiers in the longer-term, particularly when combined with the general stresses of life in the Roman army.

Modern studies have shown how ground-down soldiers can become by military life more generally, and Roman soldiers would have been exposed to most, if not all, of the same conditions, including the rigours of marching and camping, sanitation issues, and the feeling that the military institution and state cared little for their individual welfare.[52] Unlike their ancient Greek counterparts, soldiers in the Roman army during the Imperial period were career soldiers, enlisted for a minimum of 20 years—the majority of their productive adult life—and, based on demographic estimates, had a less than 50% chance of surviving through to retirement regardless of their exposure to battle.[53] They could be exposed to extended operations in the field under intensive and stressful conditions—it is noted that one of the factors which may have insulated ancient Greek (particularly Athenian) soldiers from combat trauma was the relatively limited temporal window in which they operated (Crowley 2014: 116), unlike their Roman counterparts. Soldiers may even have been influenced by the need to be seen as brave and honourable within the army, characteristics valued within both the military community and civilian society.[54]

[51] 'in cas(tris) int(er)f(ectus) ab hosti(bus)'; RIB 3218.

[52] Chrissanthos, 'Aeneas in Iraq', pp. 227–35.

[53] Scheidel, 'Marriage, Families, and Survival'.

[54] Coulston, 'Courage of Cowardice', 2013.

It is not difficult to imagine the need to keep up appearances within the military community by avoiding discussion of mental health issues to escape accusations of cowardice or weakness.

There may have been additional physical aspects to combat trauma among Roman soldiers, resulting from head injuries sustained by soldiers in battle. An exploration of the Roman medical sources suggests that Roman soldiers could be exposed to—and survive—what is now termed Traumatic Brain Injury (TBI) in relatively significant numbers,[55] particularly through concussive blows to the head.[56] Although we must be cautious about projecting modern findings into antiquity, it has been observed in several studies on US military personnel that TBIs frequently have a long-term psychological effect, associated with mental health disorders and, a correlation with higher suicide rates among soldiers and veterans.[57] Roman soldiers had a high level of vulnerability to concussive blows and TBIs—it is unlikely that their brain chemistry was sufficiently different from the modern day that they would be immune from a similar range of longer-term consequences.

The ancient evidence demonstrates the potential for combat trauma to lead individual soldiers to tire of life to the degree that they committed suicide—not due to the effects of old age, as in the civilian context, but their inability to continue to live with the psychological consequences of military life, both through mental health issues caused purely by psychological combat trauma, and those with an additional physical element, such as TBI and other physical injuries.

Why Was the Rescript Introduced?

The rescript to the law allowing certain types of military suicide represents a recognition by the authorities that some soldiers were being driven to take this action by their military experiences—and even at least a partial acceptance of culpability. But this does not answer the question of why

[55] V.J. Belfiglio, 'Treatment of Traumatic Brain Injury in the Roman Army', *Balkan Military Medical Review* 18, 2015, 101–05.

[56] Although James, 'The Point of the Sword', pp. 51–3, suggests that many Roman combatants would have been able to evade direct blows to the head during battle.

[57] C.J. Bryan and T.A. Clemans, 'Repetitive Traumatic Brain Injury, Psychological Symptoms, and Suicide Risk in a Clinical Sample of Deployed Military Personnel', *JAMA Psychiatry* 70, 2013, 686–91.

this happened during the reign of Hadrian in particular—why not before, why not after? Why did Hadrian consider that his rescript was necessary—beyond the obvious point that soldiers were committing suicide, their wills were being declared invalid, and this was causing a problem? It is not clear at what point in Hadrian's reign that the rescript was introduced, nor why the legal change was deemed to be either necessary or desirable. Did it reflect new circumstances under his reign, or was it a recognition of processes which had long been part of Roman military life, but were not allowed for until the first half of the second century AD?

Was the rescript a reaction to growing levels of combat trauma, caused by more intensive and/or traumatising warfare under Hadrian? Certainly, the late first and early second century AD was a period which saw high levels of conflict. Under Hadrian's predecessor Trajan, the Roman army had engaged in two particularly brutal wars in Dacia (AD 101–102 and 105–106), scenes from which are depicted on Trajan's Column in Rome, and on a triumphal monument built at Adamklissi (Romania), on the site of a battlefield from the conflict. These reliefs show some of the darker sides of Roman warfare, including bound prisoners-of-war, torture of soldiers, and post-mortem display of the corpse of the Dacian leader Decebalus.[58] Many of the soldiers who had fought in Trajan's conflicts would have enlisted in the AD 90s and would still have been on active service at the start of Hadrian's reign, albeit in the later stages of their career, carrying any combat trauma from these earlier campaigns with them. The start of Hadrian's reign seems to have been plagued by conflicts across the Empire, with uprisings and territorial incursions in Parthia, Sarmatia, Britain, Egypt, Libya, and Palestine.[59] These conflicts, while not documented extensively in the historical record, appear to have been fairly large-scale and, more problematically for the Romans, were seemingly conducted more as asymmetric/guerrilla campaigns, rather than the pitched battle-centric warfare which previously dominated the Roman military experience. But this was not just a problem which emerged under Hadrian, or even Trajan, but the continuation of a process which had been underway since the late first century BC, as the Roman army became more active in territories away from

[58] On the growing representation of suffering in Roman (military) art in the second century AD see Ferris, 'Suffering in Silence'.

[59] HA *Hadrian* 5.1–2.

the Mediterranean heartlands of the Empire. Conflicts in what would become the provinces increasingly moving away from the conventional warfare which dominated the Republican period, to asymmetric conflicts in the provinces—against 'barbarian' enemies who could provoke intensive fear.[60] The result of these growing levels of brutal provincial conflict may have been higher levels of combat trauma developing among Roman soldiers, both in the decade before Hadrian's reign as well as during it, with a consequent rise in military suicide rates, and a pressing need to address their wider impact.

Military suicides in the Roman army may have been a longer-standing issue, but Hadrian was the first emperor to both recognise the problem and make legal provision to address it. In part, we may be seeing the impact of an emperor who made significant changes to the Roman military system, alongside the formalisation of frontiers (particularly the building of Hadrian's Wall in Britain) and a re-focus on military training, seemingly with a penchant for peace rather than active war and conquest.[61] Hadrian gained significant military experience in the field prior to becoming emperor, as he climbed the Roman political ladder.[62] He served as part of Trajan's personal entourage during the First and Second Dacian Wars,[63] giving him the opportunity to see the conflict first-hand. He has gained a reputation as being more connected with military concerns than many other emperors (even those with strong military background themselves), despite several ancient sources giving the impression that he was not considered to be sufficiently dedicated to actually waging war as he should have been. Recognition of combat trauma among soldiers, which in some cases could drive them to suicide, and the adaptation of the law to end their total legal censure, is one previously

[60] For Roman attitudes to 'barbarians', particularly fear of them, see I.M. Ferris, *Enemies of Rome: Barbarians through Roman Eyes* (Stroud: Sutton, 2000).

[61] R.W. Davies, 'Fronto, Hadrian and the Roman Army', *Latomus* 27, 1968, 75–95.

[62] The often-problematic *Historia Augusta* claims that Hadrian first entered military service at the age of 15, early in his career becoming Tribune of the Legio II Adiutrix, and serving in Pannonia, Lower Moesia, and Upper Germania (Historia Augusta, *Hadrian* 2.1–5) before coming to the attention of the emperor Trajan.

[63] Historia Augusta, *Hadrian*, 3.2–6. Although not for the entire duration of the conflict in either case, both times leaving to take up a political/military appointment elsewhere.

largely unrecognised aspect of the changes that he made to the Roman army.

Certainly, the rescript would have made a significant difference to the beneficiaries of the soldiers who committed suicide, who would no longer find themselves disenfranchised by the legal system, and able to claim the estate of the deceased. In many cases, this would have been the families of the soldiers left behind—either natal relatives back home or unofficial wives and children. Although Roman soldiers were not officially allowed to marry at the time of Hadrian's reign, it is clear that many ignored the prohibition and formed families, albeit ones which would not necessarily have been recognised by the Roman authorities.[64] Whether intentional or incidental, Hadrian's rescript would have let soldiers know that their families would not be disenfranchised by their death in service, whatever the cause—even suicide, if that was a result of their earlier military experiences.

There is little evidence that the rescript was intended to have any effect on the actual rates of suicide within the Roman army—in fact, by ensuring that soldiers' families were not disinherited by the act, it perhaps made it more likely to happen, as individuals would be at least partially freed from worry about the financial circumstances of their dependents after death. The legal provisions were not intended to prevent military suicide, but to exculpate it, where it was demonstrated that it was the direct result of injury sustained in service, whether physical or psychological. There may have been preventative measures employed by the Roman army to reduce suicide rates, but as no indication of what they might have been had survived in the historical record, any discussion of the form they took would be speculative at best. The rescript itself represents a formal changing of attitudes towards suicidal soldiers, acknowledging that they were not deserters, nor traitors or cowards, but men who had been driven to their death through warfare; that it came at their own hands, rather than those of the enemy, no longer made a legal difference.

Conclusion

It is not necessary to apply modern psychological diagnoses or models to the ancient world to see evidence of combat trauma within the

[64] Phang, *Marriage*.

Roman army, which in an unknown number of cases led to the suicide of individual soldiers, perhaps years after the events had taken place. Legal recognition of the Roman military system being at least partly to blame for these deaths was only made under Hadrian, but he may have addressed a long-standing problem. The rescript did not aim to stop soldiers committing suicide—in fact, by protecting their beneficiaries it may have removed a barrier against it—but it did reflect recognition of the hard fact that military life would lead a certain number of soldiers to commit suicide, and that under some circumstances, this did not equate to desertion of the army. It can be seen as a formal recognition of the psychological toll of military life on at least some soldiers, codified in the Roman legal system and maintained throughout the rest of the Imperial period.

Bibliography

Baker, G., *Spare No One: Mass Violence in Roman Warfare* XX (Lanham: Rowman & Littlefield, 2020).

Belfiglio, V.J., 'Post Traumatic Stress Disorder and Acute Stress Disorder in Army: Lessons for Modern Armies', *Balkan Military Medical Review* 18, 2015, 65–71.

Belfiglio, V.J., 'Treatment of Traumatic Brain Injury in the Roman Army', *Balkan Military Medical Review* 18, 2015, 101–05.

Breeze, D.J., and Ferris, I., 'They Think it's All Over. The Face of Victory on the British Frontier', *Journal of Conflict Archaeology* 11, 2016, 19–39.

Bryan, C.J., and Clemans, T.A., 'Repetitive Traumatic Brain Injury, Psychological Symptoms, and Suicide Risk in a Clinical Sample of Deployed Military Personnel', *JAMA Psychiatry* 70, 2013, 686–91.

Campbell, L., 'Reading the Writing on the Wall: Discovering New Dimensions to the Antonine Wall Distance Sculptures', *Journal of Ancient History and Archaeology* 7, 2020, 46–75.

Campbell, L., 'Polychromy on the Antonine Wall Distance Sculptures: Non-destructive Identification of Pigments on Roman Reliefs', *Britannia* 51, 2020, 175–201.

Chrissanthos, S., 'Aeneas in Iraq: Comparing the Roman and Modern Battle Experience', in M.B., Cosmopoulos (ed), *Experiencing War: Trauma and Society from Ancient Greece to the Iraq War* (Chicago: Ares, 2007), pp. 225–57.

Cokayne, K., *Experiencing Old Age in Ancient Rome* (London: Routledge, 2003).

Coulston, J.C.N., 'Courage and Cowardice in the Roman Imperial Army', *War in History* 20, 2013, 7–31.

Crowley, J., 'Beyond the Universal Soldier: Combat Trauma in Classical Antiquity', in P. Meineck and D. Konstan (eds), *Combat Trauma and the Ancient Greeks* (New York: Palgrave, 2014), pp. 105–30.

Davies, R.W., 'Fronto, Hadrian and the Roman Army', *Latomus* 27, 1968, 75–95.

Ferris, I., 'Insignificant Others: Images of Barbarians on Military Art from Roman Britain', in K. Meadows, C. Lemke and J. Heron (eds), *TRAC 96: Proceedings of the Sixth Annual Theoretical Roman Archaeology Conference* (Oxford: Oxbow Books, 1997), pp. 22–8.

Ferris, I.M., *Enemies of Rome: Barbarians through Roman Eyes* (Stroud: Sutton, 2000).

Ferris, I., 'Suffering in Silence: The Political Aesthetics of Pain in Antonine Art', *Journal of Conflict Archaeology* 1, 2005, 67–92.

Goldsworthy, A., *The Roman Army at War, 100 BC–AD 200* (Oxford: Clarendon, 1996).

Haynes, I.P., *Blood of the Provinces: The Roman Auxilia and the Making of Provincial Society from Augustus to the Severans* (Oxford: Oxford University Press, 2013).

Heidenreich, S.M., and Roth, J.P., 'The Neurophysiology of Panic on the Ancient Battlefield', in L.L. Brice (ed), *New Approaches to Greek and Roman Warfare* (Hoboken, NJ: Wiley-Blackwell, 2020), pp. 127–38.

Hope, V.M., *Roman Death: The Dying and the Dead in Ancient Rome* (London: Continuum, 2009).

James, S.T., 'The Point of the Sword: What Roman-Era Weapons Could Do to Bodies—And Why They Often Didn't', in A.W. Busch and H.J. Schalles (eds), *Waffen in Aktion. Akten der 16. Internationalen Roman Military Equipment Conference (ROMEC). Xantener Berichte* 16, 2010, pp. 41–54.

Kasier, W., 'Justinian and the *Corpus Iuris Civilis*', in D. Johnston (ed), *The Cambridge Companion to Roman Law* (Cambridge: Cambridge University Press, 2015), pp. 119–48.

Lee, A.D., 'Morale and the Roman Experience of Battle', in A.B. Lloyd (ed), *Battle in Antiquity* (Swansea: Classical Press of Wales), pp. 199–217.

Liston, M.A., 'Skeletal Evidence for the Impact of Battle on Soldiers and Non-Combatants', in L.L. Brice (ed), *New Approaches to Greek and Roman Warfare* (Hoboken, NJ: Wiley-Blackwell, 2020), pp. 81–94.

Melchior, A., 'Caesar in Vietnam: Did Roman Soldiers Suffer from Post-traumatic Stress Disorder?', *Greece & Rome* 58, 2011, 209–23.

Mommsen, T., *The Digest of Justinian Latin Text* (Philadelphia: University of Philadelphia Press, 1985).

Parkin, T.G., *Old Age in the Roman World: A Cultural and Social History* (Baltimore: John Hopkins University Press, 2003).
Phang, S.E., *The Marriage of Roman Soldiers (13 B.C.–A.D. 235): Law and Family in the Imperial Army* (Leiden: Brill, 2001).
Phang, S.E., *Roman Military Service: Ideologies of Discipline in the Late Republic and Early Principate.* (Cambridge: Cambridge University Press, 2008).
Pridmore, S., Money, T.T., and Pridmore, W., 'Tedium Vitae [L: tired of life] Suicide', *Dynamics of Human Health* 4.3, 2017—online journal. https://journalofhealth.co.nz/wp-content/uploads/2017/09/DHH_Tedium-vitae_Saxby.pdf. Date accessed 22 December 2021.
Rauh, S.H., 'The Tradition of Suicide in Rome's Foreign Wars', *TAPA* 145, 2015, 383–410.
Rees, O., 'We Need to Talk About Epizelus: 'PTSD' and the Ancient World', *Medical Humanities* 46, 2020, 46–54.
Sabin, P., 'The Face of Roman Battle', *The Journal of Roman Studies* 90, 2000, 1–17.
Scheidel, W., 'Marriage, Families, and Survival: Demographic Aspects', in P. Erdkamp (ed), *A Companion to the Roman Army* (Oxford: Blackwell, 2007), pp. 417–34.
Shaw, B.D., 'Bandits in the Roman Empire', in R. Osborne (ed), *Studies in Ancient Greek and Roman Society* (Cambridge: Cambridge University Press, 2004), pp. 326–74.
Tritle, L.A., '"Ravished Minds" in the Ancient World', in P. Meineck and D. Konstan (eds), *Combat Trauma and the Ancient Greeks* (New York: Palgrave, 2014), pp. 87–103.
Tritle, L.A., 'Soldiers' Home: Life After Battle', in L.L. Brice (ed), *New Approaches to Greek and Roman Warfare* (Hoboken, NJ: Wiley-Blackwell, 2020), pp. 53–64.
Watson, A., *The Digest of Justinian.* 4 volumes (Philadelphia: University of Philadelphia Press, 1998).
Van Hooff, A.J.L., *From Autothanasia to Suicide: Self-Killing in Classical Antiquity* (London: Routledge, 1990).
Van Lommel, K., 'The Terminology of the Medical Discharge and an Identity Shift among the Roman Disabled Veterans', *Ancient History Bulletin* 27, 2013, 65–74.
Van Lommel, K., 'The Recognition of Roman Soldiers' Mental Impairment', *Acta Classica* 56, 2013, 155–84.

Was There Combat Trauma in the Middle Ages? A Case for Moral Injury in Pre-modern Conflict

Kathryn Hurlock

Introduction

Compared to the historiography of the ancient world, the study of the psychological consequences of combat in the middle ages is an understudied field. In part this is due to the nature of the surviving source material, much of which seeks to glorify warfare and knightly endeavour, and the lack of the appropriate language to convey the medieval battle experience in a way that fits with modern ideas of mental trauma. Medieval studies have no *Odysseus in America* or *Achilles in Vietnam* as classicists do, to take as a starting point for their debates on the current fusion of historical examples with psychological diagnoses. Approaches to this therefore topic tend to vary widely, or are usually only alluded to briefly in wider studies on medieval conflict. This has not stopped historians from referring to the trauma of war in the middle ages, or even to the

K. Hurlock (✉)
Manchester Metropolitan University, Manchester, UK
e-mail: k.hurlock@mmu.ac.uk

O. Rees et al. (eds.), *Combat Stress in Pre-modern Europe*, Mental Health in Historical Perspective,
https://doi.org/10.1007/978-3-031-09947-2_7

specific diagnosis of PTSD; nor has it stopped psychiatrists and psychologists using historical examples from the middle ages to support their own arguments on the historical antecedents for modern diagnoses. In both cases, this happens despite the fact that definitive historical diagnosis is rarely possible, for mental or physical ailments.

This chapter surveys these existing arguments and examples relating to combat trauma in the middle ages, and explains the difficulty inherent in using certain terminology and diagnostic criteria in assessing the experiences of medieval combatants as seen in medieval texts. Its significance lies in the proposal of a new way for historians to think about the psychological consequences of warfare in the middle ages by using the theory of moral injury, an idea which requires neither diagnostic criteria nor specific terminology to identify and which, unlike modern diagnoses, is flexible across a wide chronological and societal range. As the military theorist Carl von Clausewitz (*d.* 1831) put it: 'Moral values cannot be ignored in war….moral values can only be perceived by the inner eye, which differs in each person, and is often different in the same person at different times'.[1] It will apply the theory of moral injury to accounts of the First Crusade (1096–1099) to demonstrate the utility of the concept for studying historic war trauma among combatants and non-combatants alike.

Existing Approaches

Throughout the middle ages, writers showed an awareness of the pressures faced by combatants, and the psychological effect that warfare might have on them. Geoffrey de Charny's *A Knights Own Book of Chivalry* (*c.* 1350s) described the hardships knights faced, including 'great terrors' and the dangers of wounding or capture.[2] Writing between 1431 and 1449, Gutierre Diaz de Gamez, head of the household of Pero Niño, count of Buelna, lamented that knights had to swallow their fear when they went to fight, and painted a picture of men operating under duress. He stressed the importance of correct training in equipping a man for

[1] Carl von Clausewitz, Michael Howard and Peter Paret (eds, trans), *On War* (New Jersey: Princeton University Press, [1832] 1976), p. 137.

[2] Geoffrey de Charny, Richard W. Kaeuper (ed), *The Knight's Own Book of Chivalry* (Philadelphia: University of Pennsylvania Press, 2005), p. 95.

the psychological stresses of war, explaining how when 'those who practice the mechanic arts' [i.e. masons, carpenters, smiths] were kitted out and sent to fight 'some lost their strength through fear, and some took to flight'.[3] Military training at this time drew on theories of the body based on Giles of Rome's thirteenth century *De Regimine principum* and Vegetius' fourth century *De re militari,* which led to the belief that boys needed to be 'moulded' to be cold, and thus resistant to war. According to Christine de Pisan's (1364–*c.*1430) *Book of Fayttes of Armes,* this had to be achieved through rigorous training involving, among other things, physical exertion and the denial of comfort and, crucially if flight from battle was to be prevented, exposure to combat.[4] Walker refers to this as the 'physical and mental saddening a knight must undergo' so that he is trained to respond to his feelings—of fear, of despair—in the appropriate way.[5] This, arguably, could mitigate the psychological impact of combat.

In the early decades of the nineteenth century, Carl von Clausewitz made the first attempt to tackle the psychological consequences of warfare, but it was not until J. F. Verbruggen's 1954 study of medieval warfare that the question of the psychological consequences of combat for knights was first clearly addressed. In this work, he considered fear, flight, and shame in battle, and observed that knights 'were still human beings who feared for their lives in the presence of danger, and who behaved as men have always done'.[6] He did so, however, with little reference to psychological ideas relating to warfare, and without going much beyond explaining that fear caused flight, and flight shame. More recently, historians who have engaged with the question of combat trauma or the psychological consequences of warfare have largely been sensitive to the issues of terminology and problems of the source material, or sought to approach the impact of war through the lens of emotion. As Craig Taylor,

[3] Gutierre Diaz de Gamez, Joan Evans (trans), *The Unconquered Knight: A Chronicle of the Deeds of Don Pero Nino* (Woodbridge: Boydell & Brewer, 2004), p. 2.

[4] Katie K. Walker, 'Peril, Flight and the Sad Man: Medieval Theories of the Body in Battle', in Laura Ashe and Ian Patterson (eds), *War and Literature: Essays and Studies* (Cambridge: D. S. Brewer, 2014), pp. 21–37.

[5] Ibid., p. 38.

[6] J.F. Verbruggen's study was translated into English in 1997. See J.F. Verbruggen, (trans) Sumner Willard and R.W. Southern, *The Art of Warfare in Western Europe During the Middle Ages, from the Eighth Century to 1340* (2nd edition) (Woodbridge: Boydell, 1997), p. 38.

one of the few medievalists to write convincingly about medieval combat trauma, has it:

> putting into words the brutality of the violence and the emotions that it inspired was far beyond the ability and training of most medieval writers. Even modern authors of military memoirs struggle to articulate the trauma and horrors of war, either because of the difficulty of describing the reality that they have witnessed or because of their fear of giving voice to the emotions – both negative and positive – occasioned by such events.[7]

Medieval writers, he argued elsewhere, wrote chivalric narratives that 'were not simple mirrors to the society around them, but rather active attempts to champion an idealised model of heroic, virtuous courage'.[8] That veteran soldiers sought to fulfil this ideal means that they rarely referred to the horrors of war, or the fear and shame they may have felt, as the reality of war and its consequences fit neither the genre they were writing in, nor the self-image they wished to portray. That in itself could be indicative of combat trauma, shame being a feature of some of its variant forms, but it is hard to judge.

Donna Trembinski has tackled the question of terminology in assessing possible combat trauma in the middle ages, suggesting that 'trauma' could be used to describe those affects which appear in pre-modern sources as 'melancholy' and mania. She based her argument on Guibert of Nogent's (*d.* 1124) account of his nightmares, Jean Froissart's (*d.c.* 1405) of the Hundred Years War (1337–1453), and Francesco Petrarch's (*d.* 1374) grief-laden writing in the wake of the Black Death (1348–1349).[9] This is problematic because that terminology itself varies in meaning and cause: in the middle ages, melancholy was believed to be caused by an excess of

[7] Craig Taylor, *Chivalry and the Ideals of Knighthood in France During the Hundred Years War* (Cambridge: Cambridge University Press, 2013), p. 100.

[8] Craig Taylor, 'Military Courage and Fear in the Late Medieval French Chivalric Imagination', *Cahiers de Recherches Médiévales et Humanistas* 24, 2012, 129–147, 134.

[9] Donna Trembinski, 'Comparing Premodern Melancholy/Mania and Modern Trauma: An Argument in Favour of Historical Experience of Trauma', *History of Psychology* 14, 2011, 80–99; see also Ellert R.S. Nijehuis, *The Trinity of Trauma: Ignorance, Fragility and Control: The Evolving Concept of Trauma/The Concept and Facts of Dissociation in Trauma* (Göttingen: Vandenhoeck & Ruprecht, 2015), p. 16.

black bile, a physiological cause, and not by psychological trauma.[10] She argues, however, that though pre-modern commentators used different terminology, 'they nonetheless recognised similar causes of trauma and its consequent symptoms under the rubrics of melancholia and mania'.[11]

Since then, there has been a growth in study of the wider impact of medieval warfare on those involved in it, largely through a discussion of themes like masculinity, fear, cowardice and courage, and the emotional impact of conflict. In many respects they owe a debt to John Keegan's *The Face of Battle* (1983) which took Agincourt as a case study, and kick-started much of the interest in the historical study of the psychology of war.[12] Megan Cassidy-Welch convincingly argued that grief was the predominant psychological response to the events of the Battle of Agincourt of 1415, and argued that it was a manifestation of mental distress and shame, among other things.[13] Alistair MacDonald has looked at the

[10] The role of Black Bile was noted by Galen, whose ideas drew on the collection of works known as Hippocrates' *Internal Affections* c. 400 B.C., and repeated by medieval writers like the Dominican friar Vincent of Beauvais. Javier Vergara Ciordia and Mª José Ruiz, 'Psychological Characters in Vicente de Beauvais (1190–1264)', *Procedia—Social and Behavioral Sciences* 30, 2011, 2350–56.

[11] Donna Trembinski, 'Comparing Premodern Melancholy/Mania and Modern Trauma: An Argument in Favour of Historical Experience of Trauma', *History of Psychology* 14, 2011, 80–99, 86.

[12] John Keegan, *The Face of Battle: A Study of Aginbourt, Waterloo, and the Somme* (London: Penguin, 1983); Philippe Contamine, M. Jones (trans), *War in the Middle Ages* (Oxford: Basil Blackwell 1984), pp. 250–91. For emotion, see Stephanie Downes, Andrew Lynch and Katrina O'Loughlin, 'Introduction—War as Emotion: Cultural Fields of Conflict and Feeling', in Stephanie Downes, Andrew Lynch, Katrina O'Loughlin (eds), *Emotions and War: Medieval to Romantic Literature* (London: Palgrave, 2015), p. 1. Emotion is, like trauma, a tricky word for historical analysis—the term emotion was not used until the early fifteenth century when it meant political or social upheaval; Walker, 'Peril, Flight and the Sad Man'; '"Cowardice" and Duty in Anglo-Saxon England', *Journal of Medieval Military History* IV, 2006, 29–49; Steven Isaac, 'Cowardice and Fear Management: The 1174–74 Conflict as a Case Study', *Journal of Medieval Military History* IV, 2006, 50–64; Stephen Morillo, 'Expecting Cowardice: Medieval Battle Tactics Reconsidered', *Journal of Medieval Military History* IV, 2006, 65–73; Craig Taylor, 'Confessing the Emotions of War in the Late Middle Ages: *Le livre du bon messier Jehan le Maingre dit Bouciquaut*', in Stephanie Downes, Andrew Lynch and Katrina O'Loughlin (eds), *Writing War in Britain and France, 1370–1854: A History of Emotions* (London: Routledge, 2019), pp. 23–36.

[13] Megan Cassidy-Welch, 'Grief and Memory After the Battle of Agincourt', in Andrew Villalon and Donald Kagay (eds), *The Hundred Year War (Part II): Different Vistas* (Leiden: Brill, 2008), pp. 133–52.

psychological impact of physical traumas on soldiers in the Scottish wars, and Craig Taylor has similarly looked at the Hundred Years War.[14] It was arguably only in the Hundred Years War that the military leadership began to recognise the psychological consequences of combat, and tried to do something about it, suggesting they were aware of what we might recognise as combat trauma. Edward III of England (1327–1377) founded the Poor Knights of Windsor to support men who served him in these wars. In an episcopal visitation of 1378, a clerk referred to two 'certaine old knights much worn in the warrs' who were scandalising other pensioners by taking 'common women in adulterate embraces', while another, Sir John Breton, arrived at church 'late and too delicately at his canonical hours' and promptly slept through the service.[15] Edward's awareness of the psychological effect of war went beyond this care. When Nigel of Coppendene in Sussex, ransomed in the course of the Hundred Years War, murdered his neighbour, he was pardoned by the king on account of his 'sufferings as a prisoner of war' which meant he was not responsible for what he did.[16] Not all evidence from the Hundred Years War employed by historians as evidence of combat trauma has been convincingly argued. David Green commented that some medieval soldiers 'must have suffered from combat trauma (or post-traumatic stress)', and used as an example the Hundred Years War, but the case he chose suggests grief, rather than trauma.[17]

One work has tried to be more specific in seeking a diagnosis for an individual who may have suffered as a consequence of his experiences in war. In 2014, Thomas Heebøl-Holm's article on the knight Thomas de Marle, who fought on the First Crusade (*c.* 1096–1099), considered

[14] Alastair J. MacDonald, 'Courage, Fear and the Experience of the Later Medieval Scottish Soldier', *Scottish Historical Review* XCII, 2013, 176–206; Taylor, *Chivalry and the Ideals of Knighthood*, pp. 100, 149–50; Taylor, 'Military Courage and Fear', pp. 129–47.

[15] Euan Roger, 'Medieval Army Pensioners: The Poor Knights of Windsor', accessed at https://blog.nationalarchives.gov.uk/blog/medieval-army-pensioners-poor-knights-windsor/, accessed 1 March 2019.

[16] Wendy J. Turner, 'Afterward: The Aftermath of Wounds', in Larissa Tracy and Kelly DeVries (eds), *Wounds and Wound Repair in Medieval Culture* (Leiden: Brill, 2015), p. 576, quoting TNA PRO C 260/16/m5b; JUST 1/934/m3.

[17] David Green, *The Hundred Year's War: A People's History* (New Haven: Yale University Press, 2014), p. 150.

the likelihood that he returned from the crusade with PTSD.[18] Unlike the more general ideas of 'combat trauma' or 'combat stress', PTSD is a strictly defined medical diagnosis, first set out in the *DSM-III* (1980).[19] Though the criteria has been through four further iterations, its core definitions have remained the same and it is the model used for medical diagnoses. Heebøl-Holm looked at the actions of de Marle after his return from crusade, and concluded that though the nature of his sources made a 'diagnosis' uncertain, if historians wanted to look for a knight 'traumatised by war', then de Marle would make 'an exceptionally probable candidate'.[20] This looked a promising approach as it seemed that Heebøl-Holm was coming to this conclusion having taken into account the difficulty of his source base. However, his approach to the psychology was flawed. In an interview at the time of publication, he claimed that 'the only things lacking from the list of factors [which de Marle suffered] are explosions and air attack', though this was not so: there was also no evidence, for example, that de Marle suffered from flashbacks, one of the key criteria for PTSD.[21] Moreover, there was an issue with the criteria he was using for this 'diagnosis', as he chose to use those of US Navy Psychologist William Nash instead of the *DSM*, and then 'plucked the ones with the most immediate resemblance to conditions in medieval warfare', cherry-picking criteria to fit his own argument about Thomas

[18] Thomas Kristian Heebøll-Holm, 'Apocalypse Then? The First Crusade, Traumas of War and Thomas de Marle', in Kerstin Hundahl, Lars Kjaer and Niels Lund (eds), *Denmark and Europe in the Middle Ages c. 1000–1525: Essays in Honour of Professor Michael H. Gelting* (Aldershot: Ashgate, 2014), pp. 237–54; for other discussions of Thomas de Marle, see Suzanne Martinet, 'Thomas de Marle, un Guerrier Médiéval', in Danielle Bushinger and Wolfgang Spiewok (eds), *Le Monde des Heros dans la Culture Médiévale* (Greifswald: Reineke-Verlag, 1994), pp. 195–213; Daniel Lord Smail, 'Violence and Predation in Late Medieval Mediterranean Europe', *Comparative Studies in Society and History* 59, 2012, 7–34; Jay Rubenstein, 'Poetry and History: Baldric of Bourgueil', *Haskins Society Journal* 23, 2011, 90; the twelfth-century accounts of Thomas de Marle and his actions are found in Guibert of Nogent, Edmond Rene Labande (ed, trans), *Autobiographie* (Paris: Les Belles Lettres, 1981), pp. 364–65, 402–405.

[19] Robert L. Spitzer, *Diagnostic and Statistical Manual of Mental Disorders, Third Edition* (Washington, DC: The American Psychiatric Association, 1980).

[20] Heebøll-Holm, 'Apocalypse Then?' p. 254.

[21] Mike Young, 'The Use of Psychology by a University of Copenhagen Historian Challenges the Myth of Bloodthirsty Medieval Heroes', accessed at https://uniavisen.dk/en/medieval-combat-manual-shows-that-knights-had-stress-disorders/, accessed 22 December 2021.

de Marle.[22] In doing so, he immediately undermined his own case for possible PTSD. It is also worth noting that other historians have argued that Thomas de Marle—a man who strung up his captives by their testicles so that they tore off, and who Abbot Sugar of St Denis described as 'the vilest of men and a plague to God and men alike'—as no worse than many of his contemporaries in his violent behaviour, and the sources critical of his actions had a specific agenda.[23]

Examples from the middle ages thought illustrative of mental trauma have also been identified by health researchers, though with limited success due largely to their lack of attention to the source materials. The Italian neurologist, Maurizio Paciaroni, used the example of the ealdorman Ælfric for the 'chronic mental symptoms' of battlefield fright because, according to the *Anglo-Saxon Chronicle*, Ælfric vomited violently before combat, making him incapable of leading his men into battle.[24] What Paciaroni omitted was the *Chronicle*'s claim that Ælfric 'pulled out his old tricks…[and] pretended to vomit'.[25] That Ælfric was believed shows that the other men in the army were aware warfare might cause distress which manifested as a physical response, but not necessarily that Ælfric was terrified of war. The example is thus useful for understanding stress responses to the threat of warfare, but not for diagnosing an individual.

Another work tried to trace the origins of PTSD and consider its likelihood in the middle ages: *The Evil Hours: A Biography of Post Traumatic Stress Disorder* (2015) by the former Marine infantry officer and war correspondent David J. Morris. He argued that medieval conflict was 'far more personal and intimate' than modern conflict, and that the proximity engendered by hand-to-hand combat 'would have been more distressing than the act of killing today'. Yet only the sentence before, he acknowledged that it was not the act of killing but the rationale for doing so—particularly as it related to theology—that caused warriors concern,

[22] Heebøll-Holm, 'Apocalypse Then?' p. 242.

[23] R.C. Cusimano Suger, and J. Moorhead (trans), *The Deeds of Louis the Fat* (Washington: The Catholic University of America Press, 1992), p. 37.

[24] Maurizio Paciaroni and Valentina Arnao, 'Neurology and War: From Antiquity to Modern Times', in L. Tatu and J. Bougousslavsky (eds), *War Neurology* (Basel: Karger AG, 2016), p. 8.

[25] Michael Swanton (ed, trans), *The Anglo-Saxon Chronicles* (London: J. M. Dent, 1996), pp. 134, 135.

a concern that caused psychological damage.[26] And even then, his analysis completely ignored the heavy use of cross-bows from the fourteenth century onwards, and the introduction of canon in the fifteenth, which meant a very different kind of engagement from ranged combat.[27] The reality is that warfare in the middle ages means 1,000 years of military evolution which included technological changes in terms of weaponry and techniques, and a shift—at least in England—from the untrained *fyrd* of the Anglo-Saxon period, the knightly class of the high-middle ages, and the professional soldier of the last two centuries. To lump them all in together as one type of combat is misleading, and unhelpful, and underscores the problems around approaches to the psychological consequences of war by scholars without a background in medieval studies.

The Case for Moral Injury

Whatever the difficulties relating to terminology and interpretation, it is clear that medieval combatants suffered from the psychological consequences of warfare, and that these are akin to what we would now consider combat trauma: Edward III of England certainly recognised it as a problem, and sought to care for men who had been in his service. In the middle ages, however, 'trauma' referred to physical wounds, not mental ones. Since the nineteenth century it has been applied to mental injury, but with many refinements, chief among them PTSD. But, as is seen in the case of Thomas de Marle, there are many problems with trying to apply modern diagnostic criteria to descriptions in medieval sources. What could solve this problem is the use of a different approach to the psychological consequences of warfare; one which encompasses a wide range of emotions and reactions, is emphatically *not* a medical diagnosis with a rigid criteria, and is flexible depending on the expectations of an individual or their society, making it useful for historical application: moral injury.

Moral injury is a comparatively new area of research, and as such open to a shifting definition, allowing for far more fluid interpretation and application. Moral injury is, broadly speaking, the psychological theory

[26] David J. Morris, *The Evil Hours: A Biography of Post-Traumatic Stress Disorder* (Boston: Houghton Mifflin Harcourt, 2015), p. 79.

[27] Taylor, *Chivalry and the Ideals of Knighthood*, pp. 149–50.

defining the damage done to a person's moral conscience when they engage in, or witness, a moral transgression.[28] While moral injury can occur in all aspects of life, in everyday life it is resolved with comparative ease in line with an individual's personal values. It has been recognised as one of the psychological consequences of warfare, often linked to PTSD (which is primarily a threat-based trauma, with associated emotions of fear, horror, and helplessness) but distinctly different, focussing more on ethical and moral challenges to beliefs about what is morally acceptable. As Brett Litz and Shira Maguen put it, 'PTSD is a mental disorder that requires a diagnosis, moral injury is a dimensional problem'.[29] This naturally allows for a degree of variety, and as such the definition of moral injury is still the subject of debate, but it also removes the problem of trying (and failing) to retrospectively diagnose historical trauma because it is a flexible and culture-specific theory, *not* a set diagnosis.[30]

One of the key areas of discussion among psychiatrists and health professionals relates to the role of the individual in causing his or her own moral injury, versus the argument that moral injury is caused by the moral transgression of a person in a position of authority. Thus, moral injury might be caused by what the clinical psychiatrist Jonathan Shay termed 'leadership malpractice' (betrayal by a leader) by harming others; by betrayal by a group, or organisation; by betrayal of oneself by transgressing personal values; causing or witnessing unnecessary harm to civilians or their property; enduring or witnessing violence within the ranks of the military force; and the inability to prevent suffering.[31] Other

[28] MaryCatherine McDonald, 'Haunted by a Different Ghost: Re-thinking Moral Injury', *Philosophy Faculty Publications* 35, 2017, 1–16; Brett Litz and Shira Maguen, 'Moral Injury in Veterans of War', *PTSD Research Quarterly* 23.1, 2012, 1–6.

[29] Litz and Maguen, 'Moral Injury in Veterans of War', p. 1.

[30] For the debate, see Jacob Farnsworth, Kent D. Drescher, Jason A. Nieuwsma, Joseph Currier, and Robyn B. Walser, 'The Role of Moral Emotions in Military Trauma: Implications for the Study and Treatment of Moral Injury', *Review of General Psychology* 18, 2014, 249–62. Jeremy D. Jinkerson, 'Moral Injury as a New Normal in the Modern Wars', *Military Psychology* 29, 2014, 16–18; William P. Nash and Brett T. Litz, 'Moral Injury: A Mechanism for War-Related Psychological Trauma in Military Family Members', *Clinical Child and Family Psychology Review* 16, 2013, 365–75.

[31] For causes see Jonathan Shay, *Odysseus in America: Combat Trauma and the Undoing of Character* (New York: Scribner, 1994), p. 228; Kent D. Drescher, David W. Foy, Brett T. Litz, Caroline Kelly, Anna Leschner and Kerrie Schultz, 'An Exploration of the Viability and Usefulness of the Construct of Moral Injury in War Veterans', *Traumatology* 17, 2011, 8–13; Farnsworth et al., 'The Role of Moral Emotions', pp. 250, 253.

triggering factors can be the emotions (or emotional stressors) of shame, contempt (such as for the moral laxity of others), and broader social and relational stressors.[32] Moral injury manifests itself in expressions of guilt, shame, or anger, and sometimes the employment of 'numbing' symptoms such as withdrawal from society.[33] What makes it so potentially useful for historians of all periods is that, unlike PTSD, moral injury is not fixed but is dependent on understanding the moral expectations of an individual and/or their society and, once these are established, determining how they are transgressed, thus causing injury to the self.

At its very broadest, moral injury caused by warfare can stem from involvement in an unjust war. In his 2014 work on moral injury, *Killing from the Inside Out*, Robert Emmet Meagher included a discussion of medieval moral injury which argued that failure to kill in battle *for the right reasons* caused moral injury to medieval combatants, hence the emphasis on performing penance for killing in war *for the wrong reasons*.[34] Those involved in killing for the wrong reasons could redeem themselves through acts of penance, such as those called for in the Ermenfrid Penitential for those who fought at the Battle of Hastings (1066).[35] But, argues the historian Bernard J. Verkamp, with the rise of the crusades as a Just War which earned salvation, the performance of penance by returning warriors went into decline, removing an activity which could

[32] Kent D. Drescher and David W. Foy, 'When They Come Home: Posttraumatic Stress, Moral Injury, and Spiritual Consequences for Veterans', *Reflective Practice: Formation and Supervision in Ministry* 28, 2008, 85–102, 86; for a discussion of the importance of emotion in moral judgment, see Cendri A. Henderson and James J. Gross, 'The Moral Emotions: A Social-Functionalist Account of Anger, Disgust, and Contempt', *Journal of Personality and Social Psychology* 100, 2011, 719–37.

[33] McDonald, 'Haunted by a Different Ghost', p. 5; Farnsworth, et al., 'The Role of Moral Emotions', pp. 251–52; Drescher and Foy, 'When They Come Home', p. 88. J.D. Jinkerson, reassessing moral injury as a 'syndrome' rather than theory divides the symptoms of moral injury into the core (guilt, shame, existential conflict, loss of trust), and the secondary (depression, re-experiencing anger, anxiety, self-harm, and social problems)—Jeremy D. Jinkerson, 'Defining and Assessing Moral Injury: A Syndrome Perspective', *Traumatology* 22, 2016, 122–30.

[34] Robert Emmet Meagher, *Killing from the Inside Out: Moral Injury and Just War* (Eugene: Cascade, 2014), pp. 101–105.

[35] H.E.J. Cowdrey, 'Bishop Ermenfrid of Sion and the Penitential Ordinances Following the Battle of Hastings', *Journal of Ecclesiastical History* 20, 1969, 225–42.

mitigate the moral damage of war, a moral pain discussed by writers like Thomas Aquinas (*c.* 1225–1274).[36]

Failures in military leadership had a particular ability to cause moral injury in medieval conflict because of contemporary expectations about how noble leaders should behave, termed by David Crouch the 'Davidic ethic' (modelled on the biblical King David), leading by example and considering the needs of their knights, their morality justifying their privilege but also placing on them an expectation of the just exercise of power.[37] Moral leadership thus defined the elite, and their transgressions had all the more power to cause moral injury. Men who provided good leadership were consequently praised, while those who did not were criticised. Accounts of the crusades include several examples of leadership malpractice. When the People's Crusade (1096) was trapped at the castle of Xerigordo, suffering from lack of water, the leader of the German crusaders 'made an agreement with the Turks (*concordatus est cum Turcis*)' to give up his men so that he could escape.[38] Those he left behind were killed, sold into slavery, imprisoned, or used for target practice by the Turkish archers. Such acts of betrayal appear to have created feelings of mistrust, and caused moral injury. Even in less immediately dangerous situations betrayal caused harm, such as when the Armenian and Syrian merchants who traded with the crusade army were found out as spies, or accused of selling food at inflated prices, even though people were dying of starvation.[39]

[36] Meagher, *Killing from the Inside Out*, p. 106. Meagher bases much of his logic on Bernard J. Verkamp, *The Moral Treatment of Returning Warriors in Early Medieval and Modern Times* (Scranton: University of Scranton Press, 2006). See also Bernard J. Verkamp, 'Moral Treatment of Returning Warriors in the Early Middle Ages', *The Journal of Religious Ethics* 16, 1988, 223–49.

[37] David Crouch, *The Birth of the Nobility: Constructing Aristocracy in England and France 900–1300* (Abingdon: Routledge, 2015), pp. 71–79.

[38] Rosalind Hill (ed), *Gesta Francorum: The Deeds of the Franks and the Other Pilgrims to Jerusalem* (Oxford: Oxford University Press, 1962), pp. 4, 12; Peter of Tudebode, John H. Hill and Laurita L. Hill (trans), *Historia de Hierosolymitano Itinere* (Philadelphia: American Philosophical Society, 1974), p. 19; the Latin text was published as, John H. Hill and Laurita L. Hill (eds), *Petrus Tudebodus: Historia de Hierosolymitano Itinere* (Paris, 1977), pp. 35–36.

[39] For Bohemond and his policies on crusade, see A.V. Murray, 'The Enemy Within: Bohemond, Byzantium and the Subversion of the First Crusade', in Kathryn Hurlock and Paul Oldfield (eds), *Crusading and Pilgrimage in the Norman World* (Woodbridge: Boydell, 2015), pp. 31–50.

Self Before Mission

Most morally damaging could be the actions of leadership figures who put their own interests before those of the army. Shay referred to this damage done by putting 'self before mission' in his observations on American veterans, and analysis of the behaviour of Odysseus in *The Odyssey*.[40] The same anger and sense of betrayal at leaders putting their own interests first can be seen in accounts of the First Crusade (1096–1099). As the crusading army was waiting at Antioch, for example, several unnamed knights, observed by the chronicler Raymond d'Aguilers, abandoned the crusading army when they heard nearby castles and cities were there for the taking, 'in the selfish hopes of acquiring some of these material benefits'.[41] Wider betrayal by the crusade leadership, and more specifically by their leader Prince Bohemond of Taranto, is in fact one of the main themes of the crusade accounts as they express dissatisfaction at his decision to take and hold Antioch for himself, even though the aim of the crusade was to go to Jerusalem. Several chroniclers were upset when Bohemond of Taranto and the other crusade leaders (with the exception of Raymond of Saint-Gilles, who was Bohemond's rival for control of Antioch) made an oath of fealty to the Byzantine Emperor, Alexius, when they were in Constantinople. There is debate regarding the aims of the emperor and terms of the oath, but it seems the crusade leaders swore oaths of fealty to Alexius and agreed to return formerly Byzantine lands if they conquered them during the course of the crusade. The author of the anonymous *Gesta Francorum* was clearly disillusioned by the leaders' decision, complaining that it distracted them from the purpose of the crusade, and was an example of what was to come, with the crusaders

[40] Jonathan Shay, 'Moral Injury', *Psychoanalytic Psychology* 31, 2014, 186–87.

[41] Raymond d'Aguilers, John H. Hill and Laurita L. Hill (trans), *Historia Francorum qui ceperunt Iherusalem Raymond d'Aguilers* (Philadelphia: American Philosophical Society, 1968), p. 31; the Latin text was published as *Le 'Liber' de Raymond d'Aguilers*, John H. Hill and Laurita L. Hill (eds), (Paris: Paul Geuthner, 1969), p. 48. I have been cautious in attributing the responses of these chroniclers to those of eye-witnesses because of the problems inherent in these sources with that particular interpretation. Instead, they are indicative of the ways in which the writers, their informants, source texts, and the crusade participants as a whole, responded to the events of the conflict. For eye-witnesses in subsequent crusades, see Marcus Bull, *Eyewitness and Crusade Narration: Perception and Narration in Accounts of the Second, Third and Fourth Crusades* (Woodbridge: Boydell, 2018).

'fated to be misled often by our leaders'.[42] Jay Rubenstein argues that this hostile criticism was ' hardly necessary',[43] but it reflected the moral pain felt by the *Gesta's* author who was otherwise partisan to Bohemond of Taranto and yet saw this oath as a betrayal. It did not help that he was also hostile to the Greeks, as this made the agreement even more troubling. This 'ethically troubling moment'[44] in which the crusade leaders were distracted from the central goal of reaching and reclaiming Jerusalem, and instead promised loyalty to the Emperor, clearly challenged what the author expected of Bohemond, and damaged his sense that Bohemond and other leaders could be relied upon to lead the crusaders to achieve their goal.

Later, when the army was at Antioch, Raymond d'Aguilers related how Bohemond threatened to leave the crusade claiming his men and horses were starving, and he was too impoverished to maintain them, then scathingly commented: 'We learned afterward that he made these statements because ambition drove him to covet Antioch'.[45] This would have made his retinue and the wider army feel even more betrayed. Bohemond's betrayal and decision to put 'self before mission', and the response to it in the written accounts of the crusade, demonstrate a clear example of what Shay called 'leadership malpractice', when a figure in a position of leadership uses his or her own power and authority for personal and private gain. 'Of these', Shay concludes, 'careerist exploitation is the most frequent and the most damaging. The whole unit – sometimes the whole service – is damaged'.[46]

Leaders who fled from battle, thus leaving their followers to their own fates, also caused moral injury because it upset the social bonds, built on lordship, which held the army together. As Natasha Hodgson put it in

[42] *Gesta Francorum*, p. 12.

[43] Jay Rubenstein, 'What Is the *Gesta Francorum*, and Who Was Peter Tudebode?' *Revue Mabillon* 16, 2005, 179–204, 186.

[44] Ibid., p. 186.

[45] Raymond d'Aguilers, *Historia,* p. 35; Raymond d'Aguilers, *Le 'Liber'*, pp. 53–54; for the debate over the oaths at Constantinple, see John H. Pryor, 'The Oaths of the Leaders of the First Crusade to Emperor Alexius I Comnenus: Fealty, Homage - πίστις, δουλεία', *Parergon* II, 1984, 111–41; Ralph-Johannes Lilie, *Byzantium and the Crusader States 1096–1204* (Oxford: Clarendon Press, 1993), pp. 20–23; Raymond d'Aguilers, *Historia,* p. 31; Raymond d'Aguilers, *Le 'Liber'*, p. 48; *Gesta Francorum*, p. 12.

[46] Shay, *Odysseus in America*, p. 228.

her study of honour and shame in the Fourth Crusade (1204), 'At a time when personal relationships between lords, vassals and their dependents were key to the success of a campaign, desertion was viewed as the worst kind of betrayal and the most shameful, as it indicated cowardice'.[47] The chronicler Geoffrey Villehardouin (*d.c.* 1215) was particularly critical of any men who fled in his account of the crusade, pointing out when they were later punished for their failings, and lamenting their betrayal of the crusading army.[48]

Deserters often felt shame for their actions (itself a symptom of moral injury) because although a range of medieval sources understood that combatants might flee from battle, there was a general expectation that to do so was a moral failing. The *Rule of the Templars* (1129), for example, recognised that knights might flee 'for fear of the Saracens', though it stipulated that they would be kicked out of the Order if this was the case.[49] In Walter Bower's account of the Battle of Roslin (Scotland) in 1302, he described the exhausted and wounded Scottish soldiers who 'began to falter, lose heart more than one would credit, and make ready to flee'.[50] Though many works were understanding of the desire to flee battle, others were very critical. The French cleric Peter of Blois (*d.c.* 1211) and English bishop John of Salisbury (*d.* 1180) both wrote of men who acted as if they were great military heroes, only to run away when battle commenced.[51] The works of Jean Froissart (*c.* 1337–1405), Christine de Pizan (*d.c.* 1430), and Hugues de Lannoy, lord of Santes (*d.* 1456) were critical of cowards who fled from battle.[52] *The Song of Roland* praised military prowess and fighting bravely as the sign of a true

[47] Natasha Hodgson, 'Honour, Shame, and the Fourth Crusade', *Journal of Medieval History* 39, 2013, 220–39, 231.

[48] Geoffroy Villehardouin, *The Chronicles of the Crusades* trans. C. Smith (London: Penguin, 2009), pp. 16, 17, 29, 30, 31–32, 61, 92–93.

[49] J. Upton-Ward, *The Rule of the Templars: The French Text of the Rule of the Order of the Knights Templar* (Woodbridge: Boydell, 1997), p. 148.

[50] Walter Bower, D.E.R. Watt, et al. (eds), *Scotichronicon*, 9 vols (Aberdeen: Aberdeen University Press, 1987–1998), pp. vi, 294–95.

[51] Taylor, 'Military Courage and Fear', p. 136. For John of Salisbury, see also A. Taylor, 'Chivalric Conversation and the Denial of Male Fear', in J. Murray (ed), *Conflicted Identities and Multiple masculinities. Men in the Medieval West* (Garland: New York, 1999), p. 171.

[52] Taylor, 'Military Courage and Fear', pp. 130–32.

knight, but saw failure to fight well as a cause of shame.[53] According to the Tuscan poet Guitton d'Arezza, (*d.* 1294), 'shame is more to be feared than death, and committing an injustice more than suffering harm, for a wise man ought to sincerely love/ a beautiful death more than life'.[54]

A much-debated case of desertion comes, again, from accounts of the First Crusade. On the night of 2nd June 1098, Stephen count of Blois left the crusader army at Antioch and travelled north to Alexandretta. His flight was seen by the two crusade accounts, the *Gesta Francorum* and Peter Tudebode's *Historia* as a dereliction of duty, and Stephen's abandonment of the army at Antioch to their fate tantamount to the leadership malpractice described by Shay. It is possible Stephen actually withdrew because he was ill, though the *Gesta Francorum* bitterly complained that he acted 'shamefully', and Tudebode that Stephen was only feigning illness.[55] In his account of the First Crusade, Raymond d'Aguilers highlighted his anger at this particular failing when Stephen abandoned the crusaders '*despite the fact* that he had been chosen crusading leader'.[56] It is possible though that he was going to seek aid from the Byzantine Emperor, Alexius. However, when Stephen saw the threat posed to Antioch by the enemy force under Kerbogha of Mosul which arrived soon after, he chose to flee again, relating to the emperor what had become of the crusading army and telling him that there was nothing to be done.

The anger levelled at Stephen of Blois reflected the way in which his flight and neglect of his leading role were deemed an act of betrayal, which made contemporary writers and participants in the crusade question his leadership, because their anger was a reflection of the way in which they were morally injured by his actions. This was exacerbated because Stephen occupied a particular position at the head of the crusading army. At some point on the journey to Antioch he had been

[53] Gerard J. Brault (ed), *The Song of Roland: An Analytical Edition* (Pennsylvania State Press, 1978), p. 85; Craig Nakashian, 'Li arcevesque est mult bon chevalier', in Craig M. Nakashian and Danial P. Franke (eds), *Prowess, Piety, and Public Order in Medieval Society: Studies in Honour of Richard W. Kaeuper* (Leiden: Brill, 2017), p. 168.

[54] Freder Jensen (ed, trans), *Tuscan Poetry of the Duecento: An Anthology* (New York: Taylor and France, 1994), p. 177.

[55] *Gesta Francorum*, p. 63; Peter of Tudebode, *Historia*, p. 81; Petrus Tudebodus, *Historia de Hierosolymitano*, p. 105.

[56] Raymond d'Aguilers, *Historia*, p. 59, my italics; Raymond d'Aguilers, *Le 'Liber'*, p. 77.

elected 'commander in chief' by the other crusade leaders.[57] Exactly what this role entailed is not clear, though Stephen wrote to his wife on 29 March 1098 to tell her that he had been made 'their lord (*dominus*), and overseer' (*provisor*) and 'helmsman' (*gubernator*) of all their actions'.[58] Whatever the precise definition, it was clearly one of overarching leadership, and thus his actions had the greatest potential to cause moral injury in the crusading army. Only one writer, Fulcher of Chartres (*d.* after 1128), was lenient, saying only that he 'left the siege and went home to France by sea' and that everyone grieved because Stephen was 'a very noble man and was mighty in arms'.[59] He saw Stephen's flight as disgraceful for Stephen, but not damaging to the wider army of crusaders. This was perhaps partly because Fulcher revised his text after he knew that Stephen returned to the East and died on crusade in 1101 (shamed into returning by his wife),[60] and because, though he was an eyewitness to the early and late stages of the crusade, Fulcher was not with the main crusading army when Stephen deserted, having left the main army with Baldwin I on 17 October 1097, and was therefore not morally injured by it.[61]

Stephen's flight can also be considered morally injurious to members of the crusading army because he abandoned his role as overseer

[57] *Gesta Francorum*, p. 63.

[58] James A. Brundage, 'An Errant Crusader: Stephen of Blois', *Traditio* 16, 1960, 380–95, 386; John H. Pryor, 'Stephen of Blois: Sensitive New Age Crusader, or Victim of History', *Arts: The Journal of the Sydney University Arts Association* 20, 1998, 26–74, 37. Krey has this as 'lord and director and governor'—August C. Krey, *The First Crusade: The Accounts of Eyewitnesses and Participants* (Princeton: Princeton University Press, 1921), p. 131. For the Latin text of Stephen's letter, see H. Hagenmeyer (ed), *Epistulae et chartae ad historiam primi belli sacrae spectantes: Die Kreuzzugsbriefe us den Jahren 1088–1100* (Innsbruck: Verlag der Wagner'schen Universitats-Buchhandlung, 1901), pp. 149–52.

[59] F.R. Ryans (trans), Harold S. Fink (ed) *Fulcher of Chartres, A History of the Expedition to Jerusalem, 1095–1127* (New York: W. W. Norton, 1973), p. 97; 'quia vir erat noblissimus et armis validus', Fulcheri Carnotensis Historia hierosolymitana: 1095–1127, H. Hagenmeyer (ed), (Heidelberg: Winter, 1913), 228.

[60] Marjorie Chibnall (ed, trans), *The Ecclesiastical History of Orderic Vitalis*, 6 vols (Oxford: Oxford University Press, 1969/80), pp. v, 325.

[61] *Gesta Francorum*, p. 9. Nor was Fulcher particularly critical of those who fled over the walls of Antioch on the night of 10–11 June 1098. He explains only that 'many Franks' wished to escape because they feared death, weakened as they and their horses were by hunger. Fulcher of Chartres, *History*, pp. 102–103; *Fulcheri Carnotensis*, pp. 246–47.

which included responsibility for provisioning the army. The relationship between the two—leadership malpractice in deserting and in failing to provide for the army—is made clear in Peter of Tudebode's account, as his description of Stephen's flight comes immediately after his description of the starvation and spiralling prices that afflicted the army at Antioch and forced them to eat the stewed skins of horses, camels, and other animals.[62] This was something which affected the rank and file of the crusader army, and so they keenly felt his betrayal.

Other Causes

Although many of the causes of moral injury came from actions linked to the cohesion of the army, and threats to it from leaders and deserters, some were more individual, such as the shame and guilt brought about through the transgression of personal values. Though the personal values of individuals on crusade are, due to the surviving sources, often unknown, it is possible to determine the expectations of broader groups based on their ideas of what is acceptable, and to understand what constituted a transgression of those values, and how they responded to it. In modern discussion of moral injury, these causes might include causing unnecessary harm to civilians, or shame, disgust, or contempt for actions undertaken during war. The first factor—harm to civilians—does not seem to have caused undue trouble for those who wrote about medieval war. Killing of non-combatants on the First Crusade, for example, is only alluded to occasionally, and does not elicit the same strong language or lengthy explanation as the actions of the leaders which does harm. This is undoubtedly because death on crusade for combatants, as well as death for any Christian in the Holy Land at the hands of the Saracens, equalled martyrdom and thus could not be morally painful, while the death of non-Christians was not of concern.[63] The explanation for such deaths is illustrated by the death of pilgrims in Antioch. According to Peter Tudebode, Rainauld Porchet, a Christian knight imprisoned in the city, was martyred for refusing to turn apostate. After he was killed the emir, angered by Rainauld's recalcitrance, ordered the execution of

[62] *Gesta Francorum*, p. 62; Peter Tudebode, *Historia*, pp. 79–80; Petrus Tudebodus, *Historia de Hierosolymitano*, pp. 103–104.

[63] For the death of non-combatants, see for example *Gesta Francorum*, p. 29 and Raymond d'Aguilers, *Historia*, pp. 118.

the other Christian pilgrims in the city, who were stripped naked and burned alive. Though the scene he described was horrific, Peter Tudebode envisioned the screams of the dying resounding in Heaven and focussed on the martyrdom of the pilgrims in his account.[64] In another example, when the victorious crusaders took the heads of their enemies at Antioch, instead of being horrified by this act Raymond d'Aguilers explained to his readers: 'Now as we reflect upon it we have concluded that this was God's command because the Turks had formerly disgraced us by fixing the point of the captured banner of the Blessed Mary in the ground'.[65] He perhaps here sought to mitigate a morally troubling act by justifying it to his audience, aware of its potential to cause trauma, injury, or pain, because mutilating enemies did not suggest a combatant was acting with the correct intention, a mitigation which made which made warfare acceptable, and in doing so turned it into a morally right act.[66]

Most references to disgust and its associated moral emotions relate to food and drink, probably because securing sustenance was of such concern to any army, and lack of decent provisions undermined the strength of the army, a belief echoed in the works of the chronicler William Worcester (*c.* 1415–*c.* 1482) and Christina de Pisan, among others.[67] Catherine Nall notes that in two medieval translations of *De re militari* 'passages concerning provision were annotated in four of the five manuscripts', reflecting the concerns of its readers.[68] There were numerous occasions

[64] Peter Tudebode, *Historia*, pp. 58–59; Petrus Tudebodus, *Historia de Hierosolymitano*, pp. 80–81.

[65] Raymond d'Aguilers, *Historia*, p. 40; Raymond d'Aguilers, *Le 'Liber'*, p. 57.

[66] Rory Cox, 'Asymmetric Warfare and Military Conduct in the Middle Ages', *Journal of Medieval History* 38, 2012, 100–25, 105.

[67] J. G. Nichols (ed), *The Boke of Noblesse* (Edinburgh: Roxburghe Club, 1860), pp. 30, 69; Christine de Pizan, Sumner Willard (trans), Charity Cannon Willard (ed), *The Book of Deeds of Arms and of Chivalry* (University Park: Pennsylvania State University Press, 2003), pp. 40–41. For moral emotions and disgust, see Jonathan Haidt, 'The Moral Emotions', in R. Davidson, K.R. Scherer, and H.H. Goldsmith (eds), *Handbook of Affective Sciences* (Oxford: Oxford University Press, 2003), pp. 852–70, esp 857; Paul Rozin, et al. 'The CAD Triad Hypothesis: A Mapping Between Three Moral Emotions (Contempt, Anger, Disgust) and Three Moral Codes (Community, Autonomy, Divinity)', *Journal of Personality and Social Psychology* 76, 1999, 574–86.

[68] Catherine Nall, *Reading and War in Fifteenth-Century England: From Lydgate to Malory* (Cambridge: D. S. Brewer, 2012), p. 55.

on which the crusader army was forced to eat and drink unsuitable foods, such as urine and the blood of animals, dogs, rats, the stewed skins of camels, and foul-smelling water.[69] The sources report the hunger and hardship of the army in the accounts, as well as their desperation, but there is no sense of moral judgement, perhaps because this suffering was expected as part of the crusade. According to the author of the *Gesta Francorum*, Pope Urban II had already warned potential crusaders of the hardships they would face, preaching that they would have to:

> suffer for the name of Christ in many things, wretchedness, poverty, nakedness, persecution, need, sickness, hunger, thirst and other such troubles, as the Lord says to his disciples "You must suffer many things for my name."[70]

The crusaders expected these hardships and welcomed them as a way to imitate Christ. This is not the case when the crusading army at Ma'arra engaged in an act of cannibalism, when they 'cut the dead flesh into slices and cooked it to eat', in the words of the *Gesta Francorum*.[71] According to Raymond d'Aguilers:

> Now the food shortage became so acute that the Christians ate with gusto many rotten Saracen bodies which they had pitched into the swamps two or three week before. This spectacle disgusted as many crusaders as it did strangers, and as a result of it many gave up without hope of Frankish reinforcements and turned back.[72]

Fulcher of Chartres was not with the army at this point, but having heard of the cannibalism in the army wrote:

> I shudder to say that many of our men, terribly tormented by the madness of starvation, cut pieces of flesh from the buttocks of Saracens lying there

[69] For the disgust engendered by food and consumption, see Jonathan Haidt, Paul Rozin, Clark McCauley, and Sumio Imada, 'Body, Psyche and Culture: The Relationship Between Disgust and Morality', *Psychology and Developing Societies* 9, 1997, 107–31.

[70] *Gesta Francorum*, p. 2.

[71] *Gesta Francorum*, p. 80.

[72] Raymond d'Aguilers, *Historia*, p. 81; Raymond d'Aguilers, *Le 'Liber'*, p. 101.

> dead. These pieces they cooked at ate, savagely devouring the flesh while it was insufficiently roasted.[73]

The crusade's leaders were quite aware of the moral failings of these cannibalistic crusaders and so glossed over their actions in their account of the crusade sent to Pope Paschal II in September 1099, saying only that the crusaders had suffered from a 'great famine'; Rubenstein has argued that in fact not all combatants were traumatised or felt shame as a result of this cannibalism because they viewed it as a necessary act, and part of their own psychological warfare.[74] For those who were troubled, however, this was one moral failing that they could not explain away, and it clearly caused moral injury to the authors of the crusade accounts.[75]

Symptoms

There are further examples of moral injury in the actions of those who committed some sort of morally transgressive act, such as flight when others are in danger, which resulted in the manifestation of the symptoms of moral injury. When Guy, Bohemond's half-brother, witnessed Stephen of Blois' speech to the Emperor Alexius explaining that the crusade was lost, he was distressed because this meant he would not be able to return to fight, and die, alongside Bohemond. Morally injured by witnessing Stephen, his leader, apparently betray the crusading army and Guy's own opportunity for martyrdom, the author of the *Gesta* has him lament:

> Woe's me, my lord Bohemond, honour and glory of the whole world, whom all the world feared and loved! Woe's me, sorrowful as I am! I have not even been found worthy, to my grief, to see your most excellent countenance, although there is nothing I desire more. Who will give me

[73] Fulcher of Chartres, *History*, pp. 96, 112; *Fulcheri Carnotensis Historia*, p. 267.

[74] 'Letter of Godfrey of Bouillon, Raymond of St Gilles, and Daimbert to Pope Paschal II (Laodicea, September 1099)', in Edward Peters (ed), *The First Crusade: The Chronicle of Fulcher of Chartres and Other Sources* (Philadelphia: University of Pennsylvania Press, 1998), p. 293; Jay Rubenstein, 'Cannibals and Crusaders', *French Historical Studies* 31.4, 2008, 525–52, 549.

[75] Peter Tudebode, *Historia*, pp. 19, 79–80; Petrus Tudebodus, *Historia de Hierosolymitano*, pp. 35–36, 102–103; *Gesta Francorum*, pp. 62, 89; Geraldine Heng, *Empire of Magic: Medieval Romance and the Politics of Cultural Fantasy* (New York: Columbia University Press, 2003), pp. 17–62.

> a chance to die for you, my sweetest friend and lord? Why did I not die at once when I came out of my mother's womb? Why have I lived to see this accursed day? Why did I not drown in the sea or fall off my horse and break my neck so that I might have died at once? Oh that I had been so lucky as to suffer martyrdom with you, that I might behold your glorious death![76]

The detail of the speech is a literary invention, arguably based on David's grief for Absalom, but its language—that of grief, and of missing out on the chance to die with his lord—suggests this model was chosen to demonstrate a classic manifestation of survivor's guilt, one of the symptoms of moral injury, and thus hints at how the *Gesta's* author felt about Stephen's flight.[77] Joanna Bellis and Laura Slater have argued that evidence of survivor's guilt can also be seen in the work of John Page, author of *The Siege of Rouen* (1419), which suggests that 'the concept that being a war writer was an ethical burden [as they survived conflict] that needed to be exorcised was well-known'.[78]

Another First Crusade leader, Robert Curthose, duke of Normandy, has also been singled out for recognition as a crusader who may have been affected by his experiences on crusade. Both the monk Orderic Vitalis (*c.* 1075–*c.* 1142) and the chronicler Wace (*c.* 1110–after 1174), writing some decades after the First Crusade, told of the change brought about in Robert by the exertions of his long journey, and (according to the Wace) his less prudent conduct.[79] He complained that the duke was negligent, 'showed no improvement' despite admonishment, and 'evaded any difficulty with promises: he promised much and gave little'.[80] Whether that actually constitutes combat trauma or something more specific to the psycho-religious impact of the crusades—or indeed to the rigours of long-distance travel—is another matter, but it is clear that Robert was

[76] *Gesta Francorum*, p. 64.

[77] Peter Tudebode, *Historia*, p. 82 and n. 23; Petrus Tudebodus, *Historia de Hierosolymitano,* pp. 105–106; Nancy Sherman, *Afterwar: Healing the Moral Wounds of Our Soldiers* (Oxford: Oxford University Press, 2015), p. 61.

[78] Joanna Bellis and Laura Slater, 'Introduction: "Representation" and Medieval Mediations of Violence', in Joanna Bellis and Laura Slater (eds), *Representing War and Violence: 1250–1600* (Woodbridge: Boydell, 2016), p. 6.

[79] William M. Aird, *Robert Curthose, Duke of Normandy, c. 1050–1134* (Woodbridge: Boydell, 2008), p. 198.

[80] F.H.M. Le Saux, *A Companion to Wace* (Cambridge: D.S. Brewer, 2005), p. 271.

affected in some way by his experiences, his unwillingness to engage fully with his responsibilities perhaps part of a desire to withdraw from the world, a common symptom of moral injury.

Conclusion

There is no doubt that many participants in medieval conflict suffered psychological consequences of the violence they saw, endured, or carried out, and that this fact was widely recognised by writers throughout the middle ages. The language of contemporary sources did not talk about psychological injury or combat trauma because these terms are anachronistic, but the responses to warfare they portray suggest many of the same reactions that modern historians and psychiatrists might recognise as combat trauma. While using terms like 'psychological change' or 'psychological impact' when discussing the mental impact of warfare avoid the difficulties inherent in applying a diagnostic term like Post Traumatic Stress Disorder to past illnesses, they are also so broad as to make analysis of past conflicts too unfocussed. This chapter has suggested an alternative—moral injury—a condition influenced by cultural and moral expectation, rather than a diagnosis with specific criteria (at least at the time of writing), which changes depending on the moral expectations of individuals or their societies, and thus offers a useful critical framework for studying 'combat trauma' in historical conflict.

Bibliography

Aird, William M., *Robert Curthose, Duke of Normandy, c. 1050–1134* (Woodbridge: Boydell, 2008).

Anonymous, Rosalind T. Hill (trans), *Gesta Francorum* (Oxford: Oxford University Press, 1962).

Abels, Richard, '"Cowardice" and Duty in Anglo-Saxon England', *Journal of Medieval Military History* IV, 2006, 29–49.

Bellis, Joanna, and Laura Slater, 'Introduction: "Representation" and Medieval Mediations of Violence', in Joanna Bellis and Laura Slater (eds), *Representing War and Violence: 1250–1600* (Woodbridge: Boydell, 2016), pp. 1–22.

Bower, Walter, D.E.R. Watt, et al. (eds), *Scotichronicon*, 9 vols (Aberdeen: Aberdeen University Press, 1987–1998).

Brault, Gerard J. (ed), *The Song of Roland: An Analytical Edition* (Pennsylvania State Press, 1978).

Brundage, James A., 'An Errant Crusader: Stephen of Blois', *Traditio* 16, 1960, 380–95.

Bull, Marcus, *Eyewitness and Crusade Narration: Perception and Narration in Accounts of the Second, Third and Fourth Crusades* (Woodbridge: Boydell, 2018).

Cassidy-Welch, Megan, 'Grief and Memory After the Battle of Agincourt', in Andrew Villalon and Donald Kagay (eds), *The Hundred Year War (Part II): Different Vistas* (Leiden: Brill, 2008), pp. 133–52.

Chibnall, Marjorie (ed, trans), *The Ecclesiastical History of Orderic Vitalis*, 6 vols (Oxford: Oxford University Press, 1969/80).

Ciordia, Javier Vergara, and Mª José Ruiz, 'Psychological Characters in Vicente de Beauvais (1190–1264)', *Procedia—Social and Behavioral Sciences* 30, 2011, 2350–56.

Contamine, Philippe, M. Jones (trans), *War in the Middle Ages* (Oxford: Basil Blackwell 1984).

Cowdrey, H.E.J., 'Bishop Ermenfrid of Sion and the Penitential Ordinances Following the Battle of Hastings', *Journal of Ecclesiastical History* 20, 1969, 225–42.

Cox, Rory, 'Asymmetric Warfare and Military Conduct in the Middle Ages', *Journal of Medieval History* 38, 2012, 100–25.

Crouch, David, *The Birth of the Nobility: Constructing Aristocracy in England and France 900–1300* (Abingdon: Routledge, 2015).

de Charny, Geoffrey, Richard W. Kaeuper (ed), *The Knight's Own Book of Chivalry* (Philadelphia: University of Penn Press, 2005).

de Gamez, Gutierre Diaz, Joan Evans (trans), *The Unconquered Knight: A Chronicle of the Deeds of Don Pero Nino* (Woodbridge: Boydell & Brewer, 2004).

de Pizan, Christine, Sumner Willard (trans), Charity Cannon Willard (ed), *The Book of Deeds of Arms and of Chivalry* (University Park: Pennsylvania State University Press, 2003).

Downes, Stephanie, Andrew Lynch and Katrina O'Loughlin, 'Introduction—War as Emotion: Cultural Fields of Conflict and Feeling', in Stephanie Downes, Andrew Lynch, Katrina O'Loughlin (eds), *Emotions and War: Medieval to Romantic Literature* (London: Palgrave, 2015), pp. 1–23.

Drescher, Kent D., and David W. Foy, 'When They Come Home: Posttraumatic Stress, Moral Injury, and Spiritual Consequences for Veterans', *Reflective Practice: Formation and Supervision in Ministry* 28, 2008, 85–102.

Drescher, Kent D., David W. Foy, Brett T. Litz, Caroline Kelly, Anna Leschner and Kerrie Schultz, 'An Exploration of the Viability and Usefulness of the Construct of Moral Injury in War Veterans', *Traumatology* 17, 2011, 8–13.

Farnsworth, Jacob, Kent D. Drescher, Jason A. Nieuwsma, Joseph Currier and Robyn B. Walser, 'The Role of Moral Emotions in Military Trauma: Implications for the Study and Treatment of Moral Injury', *Review of General Psychology* 18, 2014, 249–62.

Fulcher of Chartres, Harold S. Fink (trans), *History of the Expedition to Jerusalem, 1095–1127* (New York: Norton, 1973).

Green, David, *The Hundred Year's War: A People's History* (New Haven: Yale University Press, 2014).

Guibert of Nogent, Edmond Rene Labande (ed, trans), *Autobiographie* (Paris: Les Belles Lettres, 1981).

Hagenmeyer, H. (ed), *Epistulae et chartae ad historiam primi belli sacrae spectantes: Die Kreuzzugsbriefe us den Jahren 1088-1100* (Innsbruck: Verlag der Wagner'schen Universitats-Buchhandlung, 1901).

Haidt, Jonathan, 'The Moral Emotions', in R. Davidson, K.R. Scherer, and H.H. Goldsmith (eds), *Handbook of Affective Sciences* (Oxford: Oxford University Press, 2003), pp. 852–70.

Haidt, Jonathan, Paul Rozin, Clark McCauley and Sumio Imada, 'Body, Psyche and Culture: The Relationship Between Disgust and Morality', *Psychology and Developing Societies* 9, 1997, 107–31.

Heebøll-Holm, Thomas Kristian, 'Apocalypse Then? The First Crusade, Traumas of War and Thomas de Marle,' in Kerstin Hundahl, Lars Kjaer and Niels Lund (eds), *Denmark and Europe in the Middle Ages c. 1000–1525: Essays in Honour of Professor Michael H. Gelting* (Aldershot: Ashgate, 2014), pp. 237–54.

Henderson, Cendri A., and James J. Gross, 'The Moral Emotions: A Social-Functionalist Account of Anger, Disgust, and Contempt', *Journal of Personality and Social Psychology* 100, 2011, 719–37.

Heng, Geraldine, *Empire of Magic: Medieval Romance and the Politics of Cultural Fantasy* (New York: Columbia University Press, 2003).

Hill, Rosalind, (ed), *Gesta Francorum: The Deeds of the Franks and the Other Pilgrims to Jerusalem* (Oxford: Oxford University Press, 1962).

Hodgson, Natasha, 'Honour, Shame, and the Fourth Crusade', *Journal of Medieval History* 39, 2013, 220–239.

Isaac, Steven, 'Cowardice and Fear Management: The 1174–74 Conflict as a Case Study', *Journal of Medieval Military History* IV, 2006, 50–64.

Jensen, Freder (ed, trans), *Tuscan Poetry of the Duecento: An Anthology* (New York: Taylor and France, 1994).

Jinkerson, Jeremy D., 'Moral Injury as a New Normal in the Modern Wars', *Military Psychology* 29, 2014, 16–18.

Jinkerson, Jeremy D., 'Defining and Assessing Moral Injury: A Syndrome Perspective', *Traumatology* 22, 2016, 122–30.

Keegan, John, *The Face of Battle: A Study of Agincourt, Waterloo, and the Somme* (London: Penguin, 1983).

Krey, August C., *The First Crusade: The Accounts of Eyewitnesses and Participants* (Princeton: Princeton University Press, 1921).

Le Saux, F.H.M., *A Companion to Wace* (Cambridge: D.S. Brewer, 2005).

'Letter of Godfrey of Bouillon, Raymond of St Gilles, and Daimbert to Pope Paschal II (Laodicea, September 1099)', in Edward Peters (ed), *The First Crusade: The Chronicle of Fulcher of Chartres and Other Sources* (Philadelphia: University of Pennsylvania Press, 1998), pp. 292–94.

Lilie, Ralph-Johannes, *Byzantium and the Crusader States 1096–1204* (Oxford: Clarendon Press, 1993).

Litz, Brett, and Shira Maguen, 'Moral Injury in Veterans of War', *PTSD Research Quarterly* 23.1, 2012, 1–6.

MacDonald, Alastair J., 'Courage, Fear and the Experience of the Later Medieval Scottish Soldier', *Scottish Historical Review* XCII, 2013, 176–206.

McDonald, MaryCatherine, 'Haunted by a Different Ghost: Re-thinking Moral Injury', *Philosophy Faculty Publications* 35, 2017, 1–16.

Martinet, Suzanne, 'Thomas de Marle, un Guerrier Médiéval', in Danielle Bushinger and Wolfgang Spiewok (eds), *Le Monde des Heros dans la Culture Médiévale* (Greifswald: Reineke-Verlag, 1994), pp. 195–213.

Morillo, Stephen, 'Expecting Cowardice: Medieval Battle Tactics Reconsidered', *Journal of Medieval Military History* IV, 2006, 65–73.

Morris, David J., *The Evil Hours: A Biography of Post-Traumatic Stress Disorder* (Boston: Houghton Mifflin Harcourt, 2015).

Murray, A. V., 'The Enemy Within: Bohemond, Byzantium and the Subversion of the First Crusade', in Kathryn Hurlock and Paul Oldfield (eds), *Crusading and Pilgrimage in the Norman World* (Woodbridge: Boydell, 2015).

Nakashian, Craig, 'Li arcevesque est mult bon chevalier', in Craig M. Nakashian and Daniel P. Franke (eds), *Prowess, Piety, and Public Order in Medieval Society: Studies in Honour of Richard W. Kaeuper* (Leiden: Brill, 2017), pp. 161–78.

Nall, Catherine, *Reading and War in Fifteenth-Century England: From Lydgate to Malory* (Cambridge: D. S. Brewer, 2012).

Nash, William P., and Brett T. Litz, 'Moral Injury: A Mechanism for War-Related Psychological Trauma in Military Family Members', *Clinical Child and Family Psychology Review* 16, 2013, 365–75.

Nichols, J.G. (ed), *The Boke of Noblesse* (Edinburgh: Roxburghe Club, 1860).

Nijehuis, Ellert R.S., *The Trinity of Trauma: Ignorance, Fragility and Control: The Evolving Concept of Trauma/The Concept and Facts of Dissociation in Trauma* (Göttingen: Vandenhoeck & Ruprecht, 2015).

Paciaroni, Maurizio and Valentina Arnao, 'Neurology and War: From Antiquity to Modern Times', in L. Tatu and J. Bougousslavsky (eds), *War Neurology* (Basel: Karger AG, 2016).

Peter of Tudebode, John H. Hill and Laurita L. Hill (trans), *Historia de Hierosolymitano Itinere* (Philadelphia: American Philosophical Society, 1974).

Peter of Tudebode, John H. Hill and Laurita L. Hill (eds), *Petrus Tudebodus: Historia de Hierosolymitano Itinere* (Paris, 1977).

Pryor, John H., 'Stephen of Blois: Sensitive New Age Crusader, or Victim of History,' *Arts: The Journal of the Sydney University Arts Association* 20, 1998, 26–74.

Pryor, John H., 'The Oaths of the Leaders of the First Crusade to Emperor Alexius I Comnenus: Fealty, Homage - πίστις, δουλεία', *Parergon* II, 1984, 111–41.

Raymond d'Aguilers, John H. Hill and Laurita L. Hill (trans), *Historia Francorum qui ceperunt Iherusalem Raymond d'Aguilers* (Philadelphia: American Philosophical Society, 1968).

Raymond d'Aguilers, John H. Hill and Laurita L. Hill (eds), *Le 'Liber' de Raymond d'Aguilers* (Paris: Paul Geuthner, 1969).

Robert Emmet Meagher, *Killing from the Inside Out: Moral Injury and Just War* (Eugene: Cascade, 2014).

Rozin, Paul et al., 'The CAD Triad Hypothesis: A Mapping Between Three Moral Emotions (Contempt, Anger, Disgust) and Three Moral Codes (Community, Autonomy, Divinity)', *Journal of Personality and Social Psychology* 76, 1999, 574–86.

Rubenstein, Jay, 'What Is the *Gesta Francorum*, and Who Was Peter Tudebode?' *Revue Mabillon* 16, 2005, 179–204.

Rubenstein, Jay, 'Cannibals and Crusaders', *French Historical Studies* 31.4, 2008, 525–52.

Roger, Euan, 'Medieval Army Pensioners: The Poor Knights of Windsor', accessed at https://blog.nationalarchives.gov.uk/blog/medieval-army-pensioners-poor-knights-windsor/, accessed 1 March 2019.

Rubenstein, Jay, 'Poetry and History: Baldric of Bourgueil, the Architecture of Chivalry, and the First Crusaade', *Haskins Society Journal* 23, 2011, 87–102.

Ryans, F. R. (trans), Harold S. Fink (ed) *Fulcher of Chartres, A History of the Expedition to Jerusalem, 1095–1127* (New York: W. W. Norton, 1973).

Shay, Jonathan, *Odysseus in America: Combat Trauma and the Undoing of Character* (New York: Scribner, 1994).

Shay, Jonathan, 'Moral Injury,' *Psychoanalytic Psychology* 31, 2014, 186–87.

Sherman, Nancy, *Afterwar: Healing the Moral Wounds of Our Soldiers* (Oxford: Oxford University Press, 2015).

Smail, Daniel Lord, 'Violence and Predation in Late Medieval Mediterranean Europe,' *Comparative Studies in Society and History* 59, 2012, 7–34.

Suger, R.C. Cusimano and J. Moorhead (trans), *The Deeds of Louis the Fat* (Washington: The Catholic University of America Press, 1992).

Swanton, Michael, (ed, trans), *The Anglo-Saxon Chronicles* (London: J. M. Dent, 1996).

Taylor, A., 'Chivalric Conversation and the Denial of Male Fear', in J. Murray (ed), *Conflicted Identities and Multiple masculinities. Men in the Medieval West* (Garland: New York, 1999), pp. 169–188.

Taylor, Craig, 'Military Courage and Fear in the Late Medieval French Chivalric Imagination', *Cahiers de Recherches Médiévales et Humanistas* 24, 2012, 129–147.

Taylor, Craig, *Chivalry and the Ideals of Knighthood in France During the Hundred Years War* (Cambridge: Cambridge University Press, 2013).

Taylor, Craig, 'Confessing the Emotions of War in the Late Middle Ages: *Le livre du bon messier Jehan le Maingre dit Bouciquaut*', in Stephanie Downes, Andrew Lynch and Katrina O'Loughlin (eds), *Writing War in Britain and France, 1370–1854: A History of Emotions* (London: Routledge, 2019), pp. 23–35.

Trembinski, Donna, 'Comparing Premodern Melancholy/Mania and Modern Trauma: An Argument in Favour of Historical Experience of trauma', *History of Psychology* 14, 2011, 80–99.

Turner, Wendy J. 'Afterward: The Aftermath of Wounds', in Larissa Tracy and Kelly DeVries (eds), *Wounds and Wound Repair in Medieval Culture* (Leiden: Brill, 2015).

Upton-Ward, J., *The Rule of the Templars: The French Text of the Rule of the Order of the Knights Templar* (Woodbridge: Boydell, 1997).

Verbruggen, J.F., Sumner Willard and R.W. Southern (trans), *The Art of Warfare in Western Europe During the Middle Ages, from the Eight Century to 1340* (2nd edition) (Woodbridge: Boydell, 1997).

Verkamp, Bernard J., 'Moral Treatment of Returning Warriors in the Early Middle Ages', *The Journal of Religious Ethics* 16, 1988, 223–49.

Verkamp, Bernard J., *The Moral Treatment of Returning Warriors in Early Medieval and Modern Times* (Scranton: University of Scranton Press, 2006).

Villehardouin, Geoffroy, *The Chronicles of the Crusades* trans. C. Smith (London: Penguin, 2009).

von Clausewitz, Carl, Michael Howard and Peter Paret (eds, trans), *On War* (New Jersey: Princeton University Press, [1832] 1976).

Walker, Katie K., 'Peril, Flight and the Sad Man: Medieval Theories of the Body in Battle', in Laura Ashe and Ian Patterson (eds), *War and Literature: Essays and Studies* (Cambridge: D. S. Brewer, 2014), pp. 21–37.

Young, Mike, 'The Use of Psychology by a University of Copenhagen Historian Challenges the Myth of Bloodthirsty Medieval Heroes', accessed at https://uniavisen.dk/en/medieval-combat-manual-shows-that-knights-had-stress-disorders/, accessed 22 December 2021.

Fear and Loathing in *Eyrbyggja Saga*: Combat Trauma in Medieval Iceland

Chelsea Grosskopf

Combat trauma in the medieval world is under-represented in the field of trauma studies compared to its ancient counterparts. This chapter focuses on the Viking age and medieval Iceland as chronicled in the *Eyrbyggja saga*, as such, it aims to establish a foundation for the exploration of Nordic literature for instances of combat stress. To avoid retrospective diagnosis, this chapter refers to combat stress or trauma in a non-medical sense in the context of the medieval period in its broadest sense, and uses current works on emotion and traumatic memory in the sagas to add context to how combat trauma may have manifested in medieval Icelandic society. This will be achieved by analysing behaviours of characters as well as the language of the text itself. While combat trauma and PTSD are modern terms, the behaviours and emotions that underlie them are universal, and it is the goal of this chapter to highlight these behaviours in *Eyrbyggja saga* and gain a better understanding of how combat trauma existed in medieval Icelandic society by exploring how

C. Grosskopf (✉)
University of Iceland, Reykjavík, Iceland
e-mail: clg3@hi.is

O. Rees et al. (eds.), *Combat Stress in Pre-modern Europe*, Mental Health in Historical Perspective,
https://doi.org/10.1007/978-3-031-09947-2_8

it appears in the literature. This will be achieved through an examination of events in Chapters 18–20, as well as the place of the *berserkir* and their portrayal in the saga.

The Icelandic saga is a genre of literature unlike any contemporaneous source. Sagas cover the stories of families and span over long periods of time, and their chapters often shift focus from character to character. They are set in the Saga Age of Iceland, which began in the ninth century and continued throughout the eleventh century, one of the most violent periods in Icelandic history.[1] The sagas themselves, however, were penned between the thirteenth and fourteenth centuries. Authorship and dating of the sagas are still subject to debate within the field of medieval Icelandic studies, but as it stands, we can say that *Eyrbyggja saga* is a family saga written in the thirteenth century by an unknown author, and is part of the larger group of family sagas, Íslendingasögur or Sagas of the Icelanders. Such sagas are driven by genealogical records of settlers and their descendants, and interactions between families, including feuds, alliances, and armed conflict of a disunified state under no rulership; Iceland at this point had no single leader and enjoyed relative freedom from Norwegian rule. *Eyrbyggja saga* progresses through time, covering the families of the settlers through to their great-grandchildren, and along the way, relates the relationships between these families and individuals.[2] Sagas such as this are the primary source of written records from this period in Iceland, and while they are forms of literature, the style and content of the family sagas are anchored in realism, unlike heroic epics or romances.[3] They do sometimes involve magic, ghosts, and the supernatural, but these episodes are seen as a testament to cultural beliefs and superstitions, and part of the lives of the medieval Icelanders; as such, in most cases they are considered representative of a more complex idea, rather than a work of complete fabrication. The sprawling coverage of the family sagas includes diversions from the main storyline, and introducing characters who egress later when they are no longer part of the narrative.

[1] Jóhannesson Jón and Haraldur Bessason, *A History of the Old Icelandic Commonwealth* (Winnipeg: University of Manitoba Press, 2006), pp. 227–28.

[2] Hermann Pálsson and Paul Edwards (trans), '18–28', *Eyrbyggja saga*, 2nd ed., (London: Penguin Books, 1989), p. 4. This more accessible translation is used in lieu of the Íslenzk Fornrit for the sake of universality.

[3] William Ian Miller, *Bloodtaking and Peacemaking* (Chicago: University of Chicago Press, 1990), p. 46.

These works were written as records of history of the Icelanders which began as oral tradition until they were written a few hundred years later. Regardless of this temporal distance, the use of violence as conflict resolution in the earlier medieval period remained part of Icelandic culture at the time the sagas were written down, though it was not as rampant as it had been in the Saga Age.[4] With respect to this, this chapter will examine the events of Chapter 18 of *Eyrbyggja saga* and the aftermath of the violence, as well as how the events are remembered by Thorarin, the survivor of the encounter.

It is reasonable to assume that some of the authors may have had first-hand experience of combat, as the descriptions of conflict are often vivid and realistic. However, the style of the sagas means that many of the descriptions found in the text could draw on broader stylistic tropes, as similar descriptions and scenes are found in several other sagas. This can make it hard to determine the extent to which the combat descriptions reflect the experiences of the characters themselves. Moreover, the focus often shifts from person to person, making individual responses hard to discern. In this light, many of the scenes in the *Eyrbyggja saga* discussed in this chapter will be evaluated as more of a testament to the author's own experience of combat than to that of the people involved; arguably the author was using 'narration as a step in the survivor's larger move to communalize the trauma by inducing others who were not there to feel what the victim felt when he or she was going through it'.[5] As such, the saga reflected wider experiences of combat in Iceland, as the existence of war poets is enough to suggest that victims of combat trauma wrote about their experiences.[6]In regard to psychological traits of characters, William Ian Miller is surely correct in his assertion that 'there was simply no reason for [the author] to invent ex nihilo the social and cultural setting in which these characters moved about'.[7]

Though relatively little has been written on combat trauma in medieval Icelandic texts, it is a growing area of research. Trauma in the sagas is

[4] Torfi H. Tulinius, 'Honour, Sagas and Trauma', *Literature and Honour* 5, 2017, 88–89, accessed at https://doi.org/10.18261/978-82-15-02955-9-2017-5.

[5] Jonathan Shay, *Achilles in Vietnam: Combat Trauma and the Undoing of Character* (New York: Scribner, 2003), pp. 183–94.

[6] Egill Skallagrimsson is perhaps the most famous.

[7] William Ian Miller, *Bloodtaking and Peacemaking* (Chicago: University of Chicago Press, 1990), p. 46.

addressed mostly in respect to the supernatural, such as the presence of hauntings or the living dead, a physical entity that represents emotion. Kirsi Kanerva has written extensively about medieval Icelanders lacking our modern concept of emotions, but rather the mind being moved, or affected, by external forces, and physical movements representative of the same. Kanerva points to words like *bregða* (to move) and *springa* (to burst, split, or break) being used to convey powerful emotions or physical responses to them, blurring the line between mental and physical.[8] Biological reactions to emotions are universal, whereas names for emotions or psychological terms are not. Physical responses, in lieu of conveying emotion verbally, appears to be a theme in medieval Icelandic literature's portrayal of this movement, according to Kanerva.[9] Where the modern reader sees emotion, medieval Icelanders saw illness, wounds, mind movements, or physical results of the 'failure or inability of the body or mind organ to prevent these external powers from penetrating the body'.[10] Icelandic culture praised control and restraint, and mind movements that diverged from this standard, regardless of type, were seen as an inconvenience and a weakness in character. These movements 'did not arise without events, things, or other people to cause them'.[11] Because emotions exist in this way, for the purpose of this chapter trauma will function in the same vein: that is, as character traits or actions that deviate from the norm and have been caused by an external force. Kanerva's work on physical reactions based on emotions is key in understanding how traumatic responses could appear in the sagas where verbal communication in the narrative may be lacking.

Kanerva's work focuses on emotions and the physical responses to them, and scholars like Torfi Tulinius address emotional responses as behaviours with regard to traumatic memory, that is, how traumatic

[8] Geir T. Zoëga, 'Springa', *A Concise Dictionary of Old Icelandic* (Toronto: University of Toronto Press, 2004); Kirsi Kanerva, 'Porous Bodies, Porous Minds: Emotions and the Supernatural in the Íslendingasögur (Ca. 1200–1400)' (University of Turku, PhD, 2015), pp. 93–140.

[9] Ibid., p. 97; see also the argument of Owen Rees against this interpretation of biological reactions in his chapter in this volume.

[10] Ibid., p. 93.

[11] Ibid., p. 117.

events are remembered.[12] Some of these emotional behaviours are unchanged, regardless of time and culture, and it is through these that traumatic responses and memory can be tracked without anachronistic terminology or retrodiagnoses.

The Events in *Eyrbyggja Saga*

The conflict described in Chapter 18 of *Eyrbyggja saga* is between two men, Thorbjorn and Thorarin. In Chapter 17, Thorbjorn is involved in a trial against Geirrid, Thorarin's mother, accusing her of injuring his son, creating a tension no doubt simmering underneath the conflict in the next chapter. Thorarin is described as quiet, peaceful, and 'anxious not to be involved in things'.[13] In a society that revolves around reputation and honour, and the expectation to defend these qualities, the preference to avoid all situations of conflict is the first signal that Thorarin's mind has somehow been moved. Anxiety or fear would be signs of a lack of restraint and control, and avoiding conflict or combat goes against the societal norm. Conflict seeks him out, though, when he is charged by Thorbjorn for the disappearance of his horses.

Resisting a warrantless search, Thorarin agrees to a door-court, a trial taking place on his property; the jury is made up of the members of both parties.[14] Thorarin finds himself in an escalating situation while attempting to keep the peace. His mother, slandering his manhood, eggs him on to engage in combat, driven no doubt by her existing issues with Thorbjorn; her zeal to create conflict may not entirely be in Thorarin's best interest, but in her own. Thorarin's weakness here is his lowering of his defences and allowing his mother's words to move his mind; a weakness on his part, if assessed by Kanerva's standards. He wavers in this moment, his anxious hesitation to get involved pitted against the shame that his mother's insults creates, but he ultimately chooses to defend himself with the support of his men. In the midst of conflict, the women, including Thorarin's wife Aud, intervene and throw clothes on the weapons to end the fight. After the fight, Thorbjorn's men leave

[12] Torfi H. Tulinius, 'Honour, Sagas and Trauma', *Literature and Honour* 5, 2017, 88–89, accessed at https://doi.org/10.18261/978-82-15-02955-9-2017-5, p. 82.

[13] Pálsson and Edwards, *Eyrbyggja Saga*, p. 45.

[14] This appears to be the only instance of such a court. Ibid., p. 49.

to treat their wounds, but Thorarin goes back into the house and finds that his wife's hand has been cut off. She does not tell her husband what happened and asks him not to fret over her. Thorarin pursues Thorbjorn's party and overhears them jeering; a man named Odd announces that Thorarin had cut off his own wife's hand. At this, Thorarin and his men attack, but at the sight of the weapons, Nagli, one of the men in Thorarin's party, 'lost his nerve and began racing up the hillside, scared out of his wits'.[15] Thorarin brings down his sword on Thorbjorn's head, splitting it to the jaw, cuts off a man's leg mid-calf, and kills two other men.

The mother's verbal attack itself is not abnormal save for one detail: his mother and not his wife is lobbing insults at Thorarin. Wives in the sagas are no strangers to putting their men on pedestals and making sure they stay there.[16] While it is not unheard of for the mother to do the goading, Aud not taking part in the instigation—and then requesting her husband not to worry over her—are reasons to pause. She seems to at least be aware of her husband's aversion to violence and hesitant to do anything to push him into a situation that may elicit a violent response. As William Ian Miller states, weak women are no better than weak men in the sagas; it does not do Aud any good to her character to withhold such action.[17] Between Thorarin being slow to engage and Aud's reaction, it certainly reads as though he has some aversion to violence, a mind movement which, as stated earlier, must have had some external cause. Between Miller's argument for the psychology of characters having basis on reality, and Kanerva's statement that all mind movements were a result of some outside force, it is reasonable to assume that Thorarin has had a negative experience with conflict, violence, or both, hence his desire to avoid it once more.

The fight, flight, and freeze responses are common knowledge when talking about combat trauma, or any traumatic response. We know now that these reactions are a result of one of the oldest (and more animalistic) parts of the human brain responding to a perceived threat. The repetition

[15] Ibid., p. 52.

[16] William Ian Miller, *Bloodtaking and Peacemaking* (Chicago: University of Chicago Press, 1990), p. 305.

[17] Ibid.

of this reaction, long after the threat is gone, is a hallmark of PTSD.[18] While one cannot expect that Saga Age combatants would have had this knowledge, there is evidence that these responses to threat were known to be common behaviours. Nagli's retreat and loss of nerve is evidence of that in this case. In a contemporaneous didactic Icelandic work entitled Konungs Skuggsjá, the flight response is documented as 'verða að gjalti' and translates to 'turn mad with terror' in the context of combat. It is used to describe the terrified reaction of the young and timid, 'gelts',[19] in the face of battle.[20] This phrase is used as Nagli's response to seeing weapons. In this case, Nagli exhibits physical movement as a result of the external stimuli of combat. Reference to the gelts in this case is just that; the author is not necessarily saying Nagli is new to battle, but rather that he reacted as a gelt. This loss of wits is not isolated in this incident. Kanerva refers to a scene in Fóstbræðra Saga where a character 'became utterly frightened when he saw men who carried weapons running after him' and though he did not flee, he froze and shivered in fear when captured by his assailants.[21] The weapons appear as the outside force that causes the movement in these men, but inanimate objects by themselves do not create fear; they are representative of combat and therefore evoke a response based on these characters' past experiences with violence.

The Aftermath

When Thorarin returns to the house after the second skirmish, his mother Geirrid asks him what has happened. He is forced to recall the violence, which he does in verse. Verse is often used in the sagas and there are many theories as to why, as it appears under various conditions with no particular pattern, but it is important to note that for the entirety of Chapters 18–19, Thorarin is the only character to speak in verse. Others involved in the dialogue are written in prose.

[18] Bessel Van der Kolk, *The Body Keeps the Score: Brain, Mind and Body in the Healing of Trauma* (London: Penguin Books, 2015), pp. 101–102.

[19] 'gjalti' in Old Icelandic, 'gelti' in modern Icelandic, both from the Celtic word 'geilt', Laurence Marcellus Larson (trans), *Konungs Skuggsjá Speculum Regale* (New York: The American-Scandinavian Foundation, 1917), p. 116.

[20] Ibid.

[21] Kirsi Kanerva, 'Porous Bodies, Porous Minds: Emotions and the Supernatural in the Íslendingasögur (Ca. 1200–1400)' (University of Turku, PhD, 2015), p. 15.

Characters 'composing' verse responses is common in saga literature and it is not expected that the reader believes Thorarin is composing poetry off the cuff. It is used as a narrative tool in many cases, and this should be no exception, but the context in which it occurs is notable. Thorarin is not referred to as a *skald*, or poet, and the verse is not attributed to a skald elsewhere, so for the purpose of this analysis, the verse seems to have been composed by the author. As such, Thorarin's response to his mother's query is:

> In the court of weapons
> they called me a coward:
> I defended my honour,
> fought, fed the eagles.
> My sword bears witness,
> put to the war-test:
> but I don't care to boast –
> bloodshed's not my business.[22]

This is the second time Thorarin has revealed he is not inclined to engage in armed conflict. Geirrid asks if Thorbjorn has been killed and Thorarin responds in graphic detail:

> My sharp edge hewed
> hard below the helm,
> hot blood flowed
> from the fierce fighting man,
> sluiced out in two streams
> from the ears, each side,
> wetting the word-dry mouth:
> my war-stroke the weightier![23]

Physiologically, when reliving a traumatic event, a few reactions within the brain occur. To put it simply, there is a shutdown in areas of the left brain and hyperactivity in areas in the right: communication is lost and emotion overwhelms. This results in a 'speechless horror' that yields constant internal sensory overdrive, as images, emotions, sounds, and senses flood the victim. A small area in the front of the left side of the brain called

[22] Pálsson and Edwards, *Eyrbyggja saga*, pp. 53–54.

[23] Ibid.

Broca's area is responsible for communication; scans of victims reliving trauma show the area becoming completely inactive, while Brodmann's area 19, a small area in the visual cortex, and the limbic area in the right brain, become active. Brodmann's area 19 is responsible for registering images for the first time—its activity during reliving a traumatic experience suggests that the victim is not simply remembering, but reliving the event over and over.[24] In an article on the function of the right and left hemispheres, Orrin Devinsky finds that the right hemisphere 'relates the external (extracorporeal) world to the physical (corporeal) and emotional self'.[25]

In the context of this analysis, the shift from prose to poetry represents the mind's movement as a direct result of speaking about an experience of, for Thorarin, unwanted violence.[26] Neither Thorarin nor the author of the saga had this technical knowledge of brain function, but the experience of the response is not contingent on brain scans or modern terminology; a victim of combat trauma could very well ascertain that recollection or a trigger evoked this rush of mind movement (emotion) and inability to speak.[27] The use of physiology in the case of this chapter is to show the basic understanding by the author of the saga of reliving a traumatic event and how it affected the mind. Taking this into account, it is interesting to note that the image-laden verse occurs when Thorarin is recalling the violent event. What can be attributed to both Thorarin and the author is how the mind is moved by recounting the violent event, again evidenced by the shift from prose to verse whenever Thorarin

[24] Bessel Van der Kolk, *The Body Keeps the Score: Brain, Mind and Body in the Healing of Trauma* (London: Penguin Books, 2015), ch. 3.

[25] Orrin Devinsky, 'Right Cerebral Hemisphere Dominance for a Sense of Corporeal and Emotional Self', *Epilepsy and Behavior* 1, 2000, 60–73, accessed at https://doi.org/10.1006/ebeh.2000.0025.

[26] In his chapter on the twelfth-century Letters of Abélard and Hélöise in 'Neuroendocrinology of Trauma in the Letters of Abélard and Hélöise', Ronald J. Ganze gives physiological context to Abélard's response to his castration to better explain his behaviour in terms that we now understand, which is the aim here—Ronald J. Ganze, 'Neuroendocrinology and the Traumatized Self in the Letters of Abélard and Héloïse', in Wendy J. Turner and Christina Lee (eds), *Trauma in Medieval Society* (Leiden: Brill, 2018), pp. 35–70.

[27] For lack of a better term, this does not imply that 'trigger' was proper terminology in this period.

speaks. Chapter 19 contains a complete retelling of the event to Thorarin's kinsman Vermund, agin with only Thorarin's dialogue written in verse. As in his earlier speech, this employs vivid imagery and poetic language to recount the events of the previous chapter:

> ...shield-bearers, skilled in war
> shook their spears at me,
> blades borne in hand
> I saw, bloodstained.[28]

At this point in the story, combat has not begun, yet Thorarin claims his opponents' brandished weapons were stained with blood. This could be read a few ways. The bloodstains could be a reference to the weapons' past and the many battles to which they have borne witness, a testament to the experience of the men who wield them. Another interpretation is that Thorarin sees blood on the weapons where there is none, but is instead reliving a fight as a traumatic response, unable to differentiate between a past encounter and the current one. He then composes two verses with a common theme:

> busy, the blade rang
> battering my helm...[29]

And in the next stanza:

> Steel-piercing shafts
> screaming songs of battle
> swooped upon my helm...[30]

Twice Thorarin attests to the cacophony of battle sounds caused by weapons against his helm, but these verses can also be attributed to the confusion of a trauma response, previously mentioned in the brain's reaction to reliving a traumatic experience.

Though the narrative of the skirmish does not mention Thorarin being struck in the helm, it is a striking remark for the author to make

[28] Pálsson and Edwards, *Eyrbyggja saga*, p. 56.

[29] Ibid.

[30] Ibid.

twice in this testimony. Because this recollection is verse, it is reasonable to consider that this account may come from the author himself and is poignantly over-sensory, giving Thorarin's story more depth and emotional value. The author attempts to pull the reader into the experience by using a familiar sound for readers.[31] Though he has an aversion to violence, Thorarin appears to have disdain for cowardice. He explains Nagli's escape:

> The targe-bearer took off
> in tears from the battle-field;
> fearing for his headpiece,
> he fled in fright
> from danger; all he desired
> was to dive in the ocean,
> to drown the fear
> in his faltering heart.[32]

This condemnation suggests that Thorarin sees a flaw in Nagli's personality that manifests itself when he ran in fear from battle.

Whether peaceful or hesitant to engage in violence because of previously traumatic experiences, Thorarin differentiates himself from what he views as outright cowardice: the betrayal of a man who was supposed to be his support. Thorarin, at least, does eventually respond to the call of battle to save his honour. The next stanza conveys a sense of loss:

> Merry the times
> our minds remember,
> the days ere these hands
> dealt Thorbjorn his death-stroke.

He mourns for the time before the murder of Thorbjorn, a reiteration of the loss of innocence that Jonathan Shay mentions in his *Achilles in Vietnam*: 'Veterans speak of losing their innocence and longing to regain

[31] Jesse L. Byock, *Medieval Iceland: Society, Sagas, and Power* (Middlesex: Hisarlik Press, 1993), p. 10. 'The medieval Icelanders wrote sagas about themselves and for themselves'. Intended readers most likely would have been familiar with the sounds of combat.

[32] Pálsson and Edwards, *Eyrbyggja saga*, p. 58.

it. They ask "Why can't I go back to the way I was?"'.[33] Towards the end of his account, Thorarin again reviles violence:

Fighting fills me
with fear and loathing.

Thorarin's uncle, Arnkel interjects that he 'must have got into quite a rage' for him to engage in such bloodshed.[34] Though Thorarin is no berserk, there is an acknowledgement that he was pushed into a loss of control by the situation, forcing him to respond with unhinged violence.

Combat continues to be something Thorarin does not care to resort to, and the author has utilized Thorarin and skaldic verse as a tool to convey a response to warfare and trauma in a way that is identifiable through experience, regardless of the time in which it is read. The break in the narrative prose for the verse mirrors the brain activity previously described as a trauma victim's behavioural response to recalling a traumatic event. This experience is universal even without having the same terminology or cultural context; physiology does not have the same volatility as language or culture. Geraty puts it best:

> despite obvious differences in cultural values and military practice and procedure, the resulting trauma may occur at any given point in time in any culture… it will not happen to everyone every time, but it may happen to anyone, anytime.[35]

The use of narrative to communicate moral injury is inherent in these vignettes of violence in the saga.

The Berserks and Combat PTSD

Chapter 25 introduces the Swedish berserks Halli and Leiknir. While Lily Geraty has done most of the heavy lifting concerning *berserkir* and

[33] Shay, *Achilles*, p. 463.

[34] Pálsson and Edwards, *Eyrbyggja saga*, p. 59.

[35] Lily Geraty, Berserk for *Berserkir*: Introducing Combat Trauma to the Compendium of Theories on the Norse Berserker (University of Iceland, PhD, 2015), accessed at https://skemman.is/handle/1946/21040.

combat PTSD,[36] this section seeks to use her argument as a foundation and heed her call to incorporate combat trauma into the study of the berserks.[37] The work of Jonathan Shay will also be used to lay out parallels between his work with Vietnam veterans and the behaviours of the *berserkir*. Although *Eyrbyggja saga* does not focus on these men as main players in the story, the way they are written about, and treated by the people around them, conveys a lack of understanding which results in fear of their unpredictable behaviour.

The *berserkir* were an elite type of warrior, described as entering a feral rage, the *berserksgangr*, in combat. These fighters have been the topic of discussion in the field, as they are portrayed in different ways throughout the Old Norse literary corpus. Benjamin Blaney is possibly the most prolific scholar dealing solely with the berserk as a figure.[38] As *Eyrbyggja saga* is part of the Íslendingasögur, the *berserkir* in this chapter fall under Rebecca Merkelbach's definition of 'elite warrior in a king's retinue' who exhibit the *berserksgangr*.[39] Within *Eyrbyggja saga*, Halli and Leinkir are said to 'go berserk', but a few chapters before, as we've seen, Arnkel suggests that Thorarin flew into a rage, which suggests a distinction between this main character's fury and that of the *berserkir*, at least in this saga. There is some argument as to the meaning of berserk, in terms of how they were outfitted (or not), but the base concept is the same: these were fierce warriors who wore little to no armour, feared nothing, and could not be touched by weapons. They were most often in service of kings as shock troops and were the closest thing to professional soldiers in Medieval Scandinavia. In the sagas, they are most often described in animalistic terms and usually treated as subhuman or servile. *Berserkir* were due respect as fearsome fighters, but instead they are often portrayed as villains. The berserk rage was indiscriminate, causing these

[36] To avoid confusion, *berserkir* will refer to the Norse warriors; future reference to Shay's work will remain in his words: 'berserkers'.

[37] Geraty, Berserk for *Berserkir*, p. 52.

[38] Blaney's most comprehensive work on the *berserkir* covers origin and their portrayal across multiple works and periods of time—Benjamin Blaney, 'The Berserkr: His Origin and Development in Old Norse Literature', *Scandinavian Studies* 54.4, 1982, 279–94.

[39] Merkelbach claims that there are four types of *berserkir* in the *Íslendingasögur*, but all types do experience *berserksgangr*. Her work expands on the portrayal of *berserkir* on a wider scale, in more sources than addressed here—Rebecca Merkelbach, 'Nature and Nurture - *Berserkir*', *Monsters in Society: Alterity, Transgression, and the Use of the Past in Medieval Iceland* (Kalamazoo: Medieval Institute Publications, 2019), pp. 101–17.

men to fight both friend and foe, a notably unheroic trait in saga literature.[40] The erratic behaviour of the *berserkir* as civilians resulted in their negative portrayal in Medieval Icelandic narratives, but it is worth investigating this behaviour and the reactions to it to see the *berserkir* in a different way; victims of combat trauma who were experiencing issues transitioning from being a warrior to becoming a civilian. This is the case for Halli and Leiknir, as they make a transition from existing within a monarchy to a relatively stateless society, and from being warriors in service of a king to, essentially, servants of a farmer's son, Vermund.

Halli and Leiknir are first given to Vermund by Earl Hakon (the ruler of Norway from 975–95) in Chapter 25, when Hakon warns Vermund of the dangers of having these men in his company. This transaction is in the interest of Vermund, who seeks prestige and to keep his brother Styr from bullying him.[41] The berserks reluctantly agree to go to Iceland with Vermund under the condition that he give them anything they ask that he has the power to give.[42] This, as mentioned above, is a hierarchical displacement, and possibly grounds for their disgruntlement while in Vermund's service. Their treatment is one based on fear, though nowhere in the saga is this admitted. Hakon cautions Vermund that he must be careful with the men, not to upset them or let them run amok.[43] This type of control is meant to keep them in line, but it does not appear that anyone in this story has any real power over them. As such, Halli and Leiknir exist on a strange scale of both subhuman and superhuman; they are obligated to serve whoever owns them, yet command a certain level of fear from those around them.

Jonathan Shay touches on the berserk, however briefly, in *Achilles in Vietnam*. He describes the act of the berserker rage as a 'godlike or god-possessed – but also beastlike – fury'.[44] He also notes that berserkers are

[40] Christie L. Ward, 'Grendel and Berserkergang', *Lambda Alpha Journal* 40, 2010, 71–89, accessed at https://soar.wichita.edu/bitstream/handle/10057/3891/LAJ_2010_71-89.pdf?sequence=1, p. 73.

[41] Keith Ruiter, 'Berserks Behaving Badly: Manipulating Normative Expectations in Eyrbyggja Saga', in Roland Scheel (ed), *Narrating Law and Laws of Narration in Medieval Scandinavia* (Berlin, Boston: De Gruyter, 2020), pp. 171–84, accessed at https://doi.org/10.1515/9783110661811-008.

[42] Pálsson and Edwards, *Eyrbyggja saga*, pp. 68–71.

[43] Ibid.

[44] Shay, *Achilles*, pp. 207–209.

simultaneously animals in rage and gods in invulnerability, which reflect the status of the *berserkir* portrayed in the saga.[45] He describes the loss of restraint that berserkers experience in their rage, and that their concepts of friendly and hostile are non-existent; the berserker seeks only to destroy.[46] In 1982, psychiatrist Armando Simón made a case for the berserker/blind rage syndrome existing for centuries.[47] Though his timeline of the affliction started abruptly with the Vikings, he suggested the berserker rage as a pre-existing concept that deserved a name in the third edition of the Diagnostic and Statistical Manual of Mental Disorders [DSM-3]. This article was published before Shay wrote his work, but also advocated for the connection between the berserker rage and combat trauma. This loss of restraint and blind rage described in both works is reflective of the *berserkir* in battle, and the volatility of their behaviour in a civilian setting has modern parallels in Shay's Vietnam veteran accounts. These veterans find themselves calm one moment and enraged the next, either prompted by a slight environmental change or for no reason at all.[48] Trauma can also interrupt normal brain function, causing transmissions to be broken, causing, among many other things, 'inappropriate reaction', which would account for both Shay's veterans' experiences and the volatile aggression of the *berserkir* Halli and Leiknir who at 'the slightest offense ... became extremely violent'.[49]

In *Eyrbyggja saga*, Earl Hakon warns Vermund about the fragility of the temperament of the *berserkir*. One such example of this is Halli's request for Vermund to find him a wife. Vermund knows of 'no respectable woman who wanted to be landed with a berserk for the rest of her life'[50] but instead of incurring Halli's wrath by denying him outright, Vermund puts it off as long as he can, which also incurs Halli's wrath.

[45] Shay does not use this term to describe Norse berserkers, but those who experience the frenzy itself; for his purpose, warriors or soldiers who experience the frenzy are berserkers.

[46] Shay, *Achilles*, p. 228.

[47] Armando Simón, 'The Berserker/Blind Rage Syndrome as a Potentially New Diagnostic Category for the DSM-III', *Psychological Reports* 60.1, 1987, 131–135.

[48] Shay, *Achilles*, p. 245.

[49] Sethanne Howard and Mark W. Crandall, 'Post Traumatic Stress Disorder What Happens in the Brain?' *Journal of the Washington Academy of Sciences* 93.3, 2007, 1–17; Pálsson and Edwards, *Eyrbyggja Saga*, p. 68.

[50] Ibid. pp. 68–71.

He becomes ill-tempered and aggressive, causing bad blood between the two men.[51] When the *berserkir* are given from Vermund to Styr, the issue of Halli's marriage arises again; he asks Styr for his daughter's hand. Styr is ready to make the same mistake as Vermund when Halli gives him a three-day deadline to respond and threatens to rescind his friendship if he is denied. Halli is well aware of his and his brother's worth as a military asset and uses it as leverage to make a reasonable request. Styr asks that the two brothers clear a path through a lava field, mark the boundary of the territory, and build a sheep-shed; no average suitor would have to jump through such hoops, even with money for a dowry.[52] This is clearly a power play for Styr to be able to control the situation without honouring Halli's request. After having successfully done the tasks given to them, Halli and Leiknir are lured into a bath house that is purposely overheated. They attack the door and manage to escape only to be killed by Styr who hails himself as a stronger fighter. This is an example of the lengths in which men in the sagas will go through to avoid getting too involved with *berserkir*. These men are often alienated from society, whether by choice or by outlawry, and there is an obvious sense of 'otherness' when they appear in the narrative. It is perfectly reasonable, then, that medieval Icelanders would be afraid or wary of the men exhibiting the berserk behaviour outlined by Shay.

Why are these warriors of mythic strength suddenly pests to be disposed of? There is a shift in reference to the *berserkir*: in the early sagas they are invulnerable warriors; in the later ones, violent criminals who abduct women.[53] In literature during the conversion period (ca. 1000 AD), they were even demonic figures to be slain to prove Christianity was superior. The *berserkir* were eventually turned into thugs and menaces to society. They appear to steal women—wives, sisters, and daughters—from other men.[54] Of course, if they were all treated as Halli, one can imagine they might resort to kidnapping their women. In *holmgang*, an armed dispute resulting in the forfeiture of the loser's property to the victor, the men must fight *berserkir* to keep them from absconding with women—often promising the woman in question to any man who will

[51] Ibid., p. 70.

[52] Ibid., pp. 76–77.

[53] Geraty, Berserk for *Berserkir*.

[54] Blaney, 'The Berserkr', pp. 279–94.

fight the berserk in his stead.[55] This is one iteration of the stereotypes of the berserk, reading for all the world like a smear campaign against these men, attempting to push them out of civil society, which as mentioned before is a clear reaction to fear and misunderstanding of the violent behaviour of the *berserkir*. The uncontrollable nature of the *berserkir* in society portrayed by the later sagas gives weight to Jonathan Shay's argument for not encouraging berserking, but such knowledge was hundreds of years out of reach from a culture that hailed them as mythic warriors, only to later condemn them as criminals and a societal nuisance. Especially in the case of Halli and Leiknir, the *berserkir* find themselves in a society that no longer needs such a military force, and neither they nor those around them have the understanding to cope with this displacement. Today, this displacement is acknowledged as an issue concerning combat veterans, and Community Reintegration (CR) is the study and treatment of psychological and social issues facing modern veterans returning to civilian life.[56] As before, it is not to be assumed that medieval Icelanders had any notion of these issues, but the trademark aggression, social aversion, and outcast of the berserkers that occur in the sagas align heavily with the behaviours of modern veterans with combat trauma and PTSD, and it is worth noting the parallel in effort to better understand these men and the way medieval Icelandic society viewed and treated them.

Conclusion

Focusing on the behaviours of Thorarin and the narrative around Halli and Leiknir, this chapter has attempted to further expand on the parameters of combat related trauma in the middle ages, with a specific focus on medieval Iceland, a society of unorganized armed conflict unregulated by a central authority figure or power. Emotions and behaviours are universally similar across time and space, and literature such as the sagas, regardless of their place on the spectrum of fiction and fact, do hold information on these concepts and in turn contributes to our understanding of trauma in this period. *Eyrbyggja saga* is one of many sagas

[55] Ibid.

[56] Christina Dillahunt-Aspillaga and Gail Powell-Cope, 'Community Reintegration, Participation, and Employment Issues in Veterans and Service Members with Traumatic Brain Injury', *Archives of Physical Medicine and Rehabilitation* 99.2, 2018, S1–S3, https://doi.org/10.1016/j.apmr.2017.04.013.

that should be acknowledged for showing the existence of combat trauma beyond modern terminology and diagnostics. This chapter attempts to lay a foundation for future work to be done both with the sagas themselves and to address the attitude with which the *berserkir* are approached in other works to create a more complete picture of combat related trauma in medieval Iceland.

Bibliography

Blaney, Benjamin, 'The Berserkr: His Origin and Development in Old Norse Literature', *Scandinavian Studies* 54.4, 1982, 279–294.

Byock, Jesse L., *Medieval Iceland: Society, Sagas, and Power* (Middlesex: Hisarlik Press, 1993).

Devinsky, Orrin, 'Right Cerebral Hemisphere Dominance for a Sense of Corporeal and Emotional Self', *Epilepsy and Behavior* 1, 2000, 60–73, accessed at https://doi.org/10.1006/ebeh.2000.0025.

Dillahunt-Aspillaga, Christina and Gail Powell-Cope, 'Community Reintegration, Participation, and Employment Issues in Veterans and Service Members with Traumatic Brain Injury', *Archives of Physical Medicine and Rehabilitation* 99. 2, 2018, S1–S3. https://doi.org/10.1016/j.apmr.2017.04.013.

Ganze, Ronald J., 'Neuroendocrinology and the Traumatized Self in the Letters of Abélard and Héloïse', in Wendy J. Turner and Christina Lee (eds), *Trauma in Medieval Society* (Leiden: Brill, 2018), pp. 35–70.

Geraty, Lily, Berserk for *Berserkir*: Introducing Combat Trauma to the Compendium of Theories on the Norse Berserker (University of Iceland, MA, 2015), accessed at https://skemman.is/handle/1946/21040.

Hollander, Lee M., 'The Structure of *Eyrbyggja Saga*', *Journal of English and Germanic Philology* 58, 1959, 222–27.

Howard, Sethanne, and Mark W. Crandall, 'Post Traumatic Stress Disorder What Happens in the Brain?' *Journal of the Washington Academy of Sciences* 93.3, 2007, 1–17.

Jón, Jóhannesson, and Haraldur Bessason, *A History of the Old Icelandic Commonwealth* (Winnipeg: University of Manitoba Press, 2006).

Kanerva, Kirsi, 'Porous Bodies, Porous Minds: Emotions and the Supernatural in the Íslendingasögur (Ca. 1200–1400)' (University of Turku, PhD, 2015).

Larson, Laurence Marcellus (trans), *Konungs Skuggsjá Speculum Regale* (New York: The American-Scandinavian Foundation, 1917).

Merkelbach, Rebecca, 'Nature and Nurture - *Berserkir*', *Monsters in Society: Alterity, Transgression, and the Use of the Past in Medieval Iceland* (Kalamazoo: Medieval Institute Publications, 2019), pp. 101–17.

Miller, William Ian, *Bloodtaking and Peacemaking* (Chicago: University of Chicago Press, 1990).
Pálsson, Hermann, and Paul Edwards (trans), '18-28', *Eyrbyggja Saga*, 2nd ed. (London: Penguin Books, 1989).
Ruiter, Keith, 'Berserks Behaving Badly: Manipulating Normative Expectations in *Eyrbyggja Saga*', in Roland Scheel (ed), *Narrating Law and Laws of Narration in Medieval Scandinavia* (Berlin, Boston: De Gruyter, 2020), pp. 171–84, accessed at https://doi.org/10.1515/9783110661811-008.
Scott, Forest S., 'The Woman Who Knows: Female Characters in *Eyrbyggja Saga*', *Parergon* 3, 1985, 73–91.
Shay, Jonathan, *Achilles in Vietnam: Combat Trauma and the Undoing of Character* (New York: Scribner, 2003).
Simón, Armando, 'The Berserker/Blind Rage Syndrome as a Potentially New Diagnostic Category for the DSM-III', Psychological Reports 60.1, 1987, 131–35.
Sturluson, Snorri, and Lee M. Hollander, 'Heimskringla: History of the Kings of Norway', in *Heimskringla: History of the Kings of Norway* (Austin: University of Texas Press, 1964).
Tulinius, Torfi H., 'Honour, Sagas and Trauma', *Literature and Honour* 5, 2017, 88–89, accessed at https://doi.org/10.18261/978-82-15-02955-9-2017-5.
Van der Kolk, Bessel, *The Body Keeps the Score: Brain, Mind and Body in the Healing of Trauma* (London: Penguin Books, 2015).
Ward, Christie L., 'Grendel and Berserkergang', *Lambda Alpha Journal* 40, 2010, 71–89, accessed at https://soar.wichita.edu/bitstream/handle/10057/3891/LAJ_2010_71-89.pdf?sequence=1.
Zoëga, Geir T., 'Springa', *A Concise Dictionary of Old Icelandic* (Toronto: University of Toronto Press, 2004).

Understandings of Adversity and Resilience Amongst Women and Children During the Seventeenth-Century British Civil Wars

Ismini Pells

The ramifications of the British Civil Wars of 1642–1651 were not confined to male combatants. As the king and Parliament fought over the extent of their powers in the government of England, some women and what might be today termed 'child soldiers' joined the ranks of the armies on both sides.[1] Many more women and children took on supporting roles that were vital to the day-to-day functioning of the various armed forces. Women supplied and prepared food, laundered and mended clothes, and tended the sick, infirm and wounded. Boys acted as pages, servants or apprentices to military personnel, whilst girls assisted adult women in the field or garrison as maids.[2] Across the British Isles, as the war in England and Wales interconnected with a wider series of conflicts that

[1] Mark Stoyle, '"Give mee a Souldier's Coat": Female Cross-Dressing During the English Civil War', *History* 103.354, 2018, 5–26; Ismini Pells, 'Children, Childhood and Armies During the British Civil Wars', forthcoming.

[2] Ibid.

I. Pells (✉)
University of Oxford, Oxford, UK
e-mail: ismini.pells@conted.ox.ac.uk

O. Rees et al. (eds.), *Combat Stress in Pre-modern Europe*, Mental Health in Historical Perspective,
https://doi.org/10.1007/978-3-031-09947-2_9

included Scotland and Ireland, numerous women and children were first-hand witnesses to the fighting as the defenders of fortified strongholds or as inhabitants of garrisoned and besieged towns.[3] The consequences of the war were not brought to an end either by the execution of King Charles I in 1649, the establishment of the Commonwealth government (1649–1653) or Cromwellian Protectorate (1653–1659), or the Restoration of Charles II to the throne in 1660. It is estimated that a greater percentage of the population died as a result of the Civil Wars than both World Wars, meaning that many women and children lived with bereavement and impoverishment through the deaths of husbands and fathers on campaign.[4]

The catastrophic scale of the Civil Wars has prompted a recent interest in its psychological impact.[5] However, the focus of these studies has remained firmly fixed on male veterans, whilst the psychological responses of women and children have largely been neglected. There are, of course, numerous methodological problems associated with identifying and analyzing psychological reactions in the past, but it is worth noting the irony of the fact that the debate has continued to centre on the concept of trauma, and post-traumatic stress disorder (PTSD) in particular. Practitioners working in modern post-conflict countries considered the debate over the validity of the concept of PTSD and trauma-focused interventions as rather dated back in 2007, pointing out that the then current UICEF 'good practice' guidelines for psychosocial care and

[3] For example, Edward Halsall, 'A Journal of the Siege of Lathom House', in Julius Hutchinson (ed), *Memoirs of the Life of Colonel Hutchinson* (London: Henry G. Bohn, 1848), pp. 491–518; Eliot Warburton, *Memoirs of Prince Rupert and the Cavaliers* (London: Richard Bentley, 1849), vol I, p. 529.

[4] Ian Gentles, *The English Revolution and the Wars in the Three Kingdoms, 1638–1652* (London: Pearson Education, 2007), pp. 436–37.

[5] David Appleby, 'Veteran Politics in Restoration England, 1660–1670,' *The Seventeenth Century* 28, 2013, 334; Ismini Pells, 'Soliciting Sympathy: The Search for Psychological Trauma in Seventeenth-Century English Civil War Maimed Soldiers' Petitions', in Erin Peters and Cynthia Richards (eds), *Early Modern Trauma: Europe and the Atlantic World* (Lincoln, NE: University of Nebraska Press, 2021), pp. 129–50; Erin Peters, "Trauma Narratives of the English Civil War," *Journal for Early Modern Cultural Studies* 16, 2016, 78–94; Erin Peters, "The Deep Staines These Wars Will Leave Behind': Psychological Wounds and Curative Methods in the English Civil Wars', in David Appleby and Andrew Hopper (eds), *Battle-Scarred: Mortality, Medical Care and Military Welfare in the British Civil Wars* (Manchester: Manchester University Press, 2018), pp. 156–73.

support did not advocate trauma healing as a starting point.[6] Thus, historical scholarship too must move beyond its preoccupation with the debates surrounding the validity of historical trauma and instead focus on the ways individuals in the past mitigated the influence of violence and disruption.

Psychiatrists such as Derek Summerfield and Patrick Bracken have argued that there is a tendency in modern society to reduce complex experiences to the single category of 'trauma'.[7] Framing problems with thoughts, emotions, behaviours and relationships from a narrow medical perspective 'can be profoundly disempowering and stigmatizing'.[8] Western psychological frameworks are seen as 'having universal validity' and characterisations of childhood trauma are based on a Western vision of childhood that may not be applicable to all parts of the world.[9] Instead, Summerfield maintained that 'Every culture has its own reserves of psychological knowledge, range of attributions to assign to adverse experience, and forms of accommodation, struggle and help-seeking'.[10] Western psychological frameworks have been criticized in their attitudes towards children in particular, as they have been based on constructions of childhood that emphasize innocence, vulnerability and dependence, and where children are viewed 'as passive victims and not active survivors'.[11] Several modern practitioners have questioned if children are inherently vulnerable and if warfare is invariably bad for them.[12] A wealth of evidence has paid tribute to their remarkable resilience and the differing ways they have sought to overcome adversity.[13]

A study of adversity and resilience amongst women and children from an historical perspective may be useful for a number of reasons. Firstly,

[6] Linda Dowdney, 'Trauma, Resilience and Cultural Hearing: How Do We Move Forward?' *Child Soldiers International Psychosocial Paper*, 2007, 2–3.

[7] Derek Summerfield, 'Childhood, War, Refugeedom and "Trauma": Three Core Questions for Mental Health Professionals', *Journal of Transcultural Psychiatry* 37, 2000, 423, 427; Patrick Bracken, *Trauma: Culture, Meaning and Philosophy* (London: Whurr, 2002), p. 3.

[8] Ibid., p. 4.

[9] Summerfield, 'Childhood, War, Refugeedom and "Trauma"', pp. 421, 427.

[10] Ibid., pp. 421–22.

[11] Ibid., pp. 424–25.

[12] Jo Boyden, 'Children Under Fire: Challenging Assumptions About Children's Resilience', *Children, Youth and Environments* 13, 2003, 14.

[13] Ibid., p. 9.

Bracken identified historians as one of the key players in helping to recognize the importance of cultural relevance in understanding reactions to adverse experiences.[14] Furthermore, gender and age have been shown to be pivotal factors determining an individual's susceptibility to risk and the survival strategies available to them.[15] Simultaneously, Western psychological frameworks have been criticized for perceiving childhood as a natural and distinct phase of the human lifecycle instead of 'a diverse, shifting category that follows certain biological sequences, and responds to the cultural and social environment, genetic heritage, personal agency and economic and political circumstance'.[16] Historians have long been mindful of how gender differences were manifested in experiences in the past, and also that childhood is not a universal reality but a mutable state of being that is defined according to a variety of cultural economic contexts.[17]

Resilience, broadly defined as 'positive adaptation despite adversity', has been a popular topic since the beginning of the twenty-first century.[18] Paul Garrett even contended that '"Resilience" is now a "keyword" and a focal concern within the academic literature of social work... and academics are falling over themselves to conduct research on it'.[19] The popularity of feel-good tales of triumph over adversity is understandable, especially in the media, trade literature and contemporary discourse.[20] The concept of resilience has been to some extent welcomed in development studies because it recognizes individuals, especially the young, 'as competent social agents rather than inherently vulnerable beings that

14 Bracken, *Trauma*, p. 4.

15 Boyden, 'Children Under Fire', pp. 10–12.

16 Ibid., pp. 2, 9.

17 For examples of this pertaining to the Civil Wars, see: Ann Hughes, *Gender and the English Revolution* (Abingdon: Routledge, 2012) and Pells, 'Children, Childhood and Armies During the British Civil Wars'.

18 Dorothy Bottrell, 'Responsibilised Resilience? Reworking Neoliberal Social Policy Texts', *M/C Journal* 16, 2013, http://journal.media-culture.org.au/index.php/mcjournal/article/view/708, accessed 9 May 2019.

19 Paul Garrett, 'Questioning Tales of "Ordinary Magic": "Resilience" and Neo-Liberal Reasoning', *British Journal of Social Work* 46, 2016, 1909–10.

20 Elizabeth Cooper and Jo Boyden, 'Questioning the Power of Resilience: Are Children Up to the Task of Disrupting the Transmission of Poverty?' *Chronic Poverty Research Centre Working Paper*, 73, 2007, 1, http://dx.doi.org/10.2139/ssrn.1753009, accessed 9 May 2019.

are wholly dependent on others for their survival'.[21] However, resilience research has not been without its problems. Critics have noted that studies tend to emphasize individual agency but fail to acknowledge the influence of both genetics and environmental factors, the latter including broader socio-economic structures.[22] This can potentially result in negative effects. Firstly, the emphasis on individual agency can be used to absolve the state and other powerful actors from the moral responsibility to provide the resources which can be used to overcome adversity, a criticism particularly propounded by Michael Ungar.[23] It has not escaped scholars' attention that the popularity of resilience discourse has coincided with a period of austerity and neoliberal agendas to roll back the provisions of the welfare state.[24] Secondly, ignoring broader structures can obscure socio-economic inequalities 'that are fundamental barriers to the wellbeing of the poor and blames and penalizes them for what are intertextually deemed to be their failings, deficits and unhealthy dependencies'.[25] Finally, resilience studies sometime risk losing sight of the human suffering that may still be experienced in overcoming adversity.[26]

At the heart of the problems surrounding resilience research is the fact that, as Jo Boyden and Elizabeth Cooper explained, 'Scholarly debates have yet to produce clarity on the definition, locus, determinants, mediating and moderating factors and outcomes of resilience'.[27] Indeed, most researchers settle for offering 'only very general indicators of positive adaptation', which is justified on the grounds of cultural sensitivity.[28] Identifying what constitutes an adverse situation and a positive adaptation is predicated on values, interests and assumptions, which may not be

[21] Ibid., pp. 3–4.

[22] Ibid., pp. 4–5.

[23] Ibid., p. 5; Dowdney, 'Trauma, Resilience and Cultural Hearing', p. 2; Michael Ungar, 'Introduction: Resilience Across Cultures and Contexts', in Michael Ungar (ed), *Handbook for Working with Children and Youth: Pathways to Resilience Across Cultures and Contexts* (London: Sage, 2005), p. xvi.

[24] Garrett, 'Questioning Tales of "Ordinary Magic"', pp. 1918–21; Bottrell, 'Responsibilised Resilience?

[25] Ibid.

[26] Ibid.

[27] Cooper and Boyden, 'Questioning the Power of Resilience', p. 6.

[28] Ibid., p. 7.

shared between the researcher and their subject(s).[29] Moreover, responses which seem to represent a positive adaptation at one time may result in later negative effects. For example, emotional numbing may assist individuals in overcoming adversity but may later reduce their capability of interacting with others.[30]

Thus, it seems that a study of adversity and resilience in historical contexts may be as fraught with danger as any study of trauma. The matter is further complicated by the nature of the available primary material. Surviving sources written by women are less numerous than those composed by men, whilst sources scripted by children are even scanter still. The words and activities of women and children were often recorded by others, but these were noted according to the author's own perceptions or purposes, and often with a specific audience in mind. In addition, the long-term perspective of a particular experience is often absent from most sources. Nevertheless, although the responses recorded in the sources must be treated cautiously, these responses will have been shaped by the social, economic and cultural contexts these women and children shared and negotiated with those who wrote about them.[31] If we are to accept that resilience is contingent on the convergence of genetics, cultural factors and socio-economic structures, then a historical perspective can be useful in highlighting and developing knowledge about at least the relativism of cultural factors and importance of socio-economic structures to an individual's survival strategy in the aftermath of conflict.

Following the advice of Boyden and Cooper, this study will relinquish the metaphor of resilience and focus on the ways in which women and children adapted their lives in response to the upheavals of the Civil Wars.[32] It will avoid value judgements as to how far these individuals 'succeeded' in 'overcoming adversity' but instead demonstrate how the options available to them varied according to differences of age, socio-economic background and gender. The survival strategies adopted will be examined firmly in the context of what is known about contemporary social norms, values, dynamics and power structures of the pre-conflict society, in order to gain a deeper understanding of the specific ways the

[29] Ibid., pp. 6–7.

[30] Ibid., p. 7.

[31] Boyden, 'Children Under Fire', pp. 12–14.

[32] Cooper and Boyden, 'Questioning the Power of Resilience', p. 12.

Civil Wars impacted upon women and children.[33] This analysis will be structured around four key themes: religion, family and community, political engagement, and poverty and employment. It will recognize that women may not have only responded to the Civil Wars in different ways to men, and children responded in different ways to adults, but women and children may have responded in differing ways amongst themselves. Throughout, sensitivity will be paid to the problems of the source material and the aim of the study is to stimulate further debate in the field, rather than offer concrete conclusions.

Religion

Religious faith seems to have been a common source of comfort for many women and children in the Civil Wars who faced life-threatening situations or human loss. The sixteen-year-old Robert Harley was the younger son of the prominent parliamentarian gentleman Sir Robert Harley and his wife Brilliana of Brampton Bryan in Herefordshire. He joined Sir William Waller's parliamentarian army as a lieutenant in his elder brother Edwards's troop of horse.[34] It was not unusual for youths to join an army at his age, especially amongst sons of the gentry and nobility, but the age at which it was considered appropriate to take up arms in the Civil Wars was debated and Harley would have been considered too young by some.[35] Writing to Edward in 1644, Robert openly acknowledged the 'terror' and 'fear' that preceded engagements. Yet, he was adamant of 'God's mercy towards us' and that the battle of Cheriton would have been lost 'if God had not wonderfully shewed himselfe'.[36] Likewise, Joseph Lister apparently described an incident in Pudsey Church, Yorkshire, which he witnessed as a fifteen-year-old when 'the people's hearts failed them' at news that the Irish had landed in Lancashire but the minister composed them by putting 'himself and them into the hands of Almighty

[33] Boyden, 'Children Under Fire', p. 7.

[34] Stephen Roberts, ed., 'Surnames Beginning 'H', *The Cromwell Association Online Directory of Parliamentarian Army Officers* (2017), https://www.british-history.ac.uk/no-series/cromwell-army-officers/surnames-h, accessed 19 February 2018.

[35] Pells, 'Children, Childhood and Armies During the British Civil Wars'.

[36] *The Manuscripts of His Grace the Duke of Portland: Preserved at Welbeck Abbey* (10 vols, London: H.M.S.O., 1891–1931), vol III, pp. 106, 108.

God'.[37] When Prince Rupert's royalist army stormed Liverpool in June 1644, one woman known only by her initials, M. W., had her husband and one child killed before her eyes. She and her remaining child—who was merely five years' old—were stripped and wounded. Nevertheless, for this woman 'our cause was God's and our enemies [were] popish rebels;... so I took it patiently... and in this confidence did rejoice with my wounded child and little daughter, in a barn where we were put, having gotten a piece of an old Bible'.[38]

It may hardly seem surprising that the Pudsey minister calmed his congregation with religious reassurances or that Harley, raised in a famously puritan family (a member of which he was, of course, writing to), attributed his preservation to the Almighty. Similarly, M. W.'s story was only documented for posterity when she related it to an Independent congregation in London. It cannot be ruled out that she tailored her recollections to her audience or that these were embellished by the recording minister for his own instructional purposes. However, when faced with the religiously saturated language of the seventeenth century, it is easy for historians to forget that these were sincerely held beliefs. Both Bracken and Summerfield highlighted the continued importance of religion and spirituality to making sense of life in many parts of the modern world.[39] Summerfield warned that medical and psychological terminology have replaced religious vocabulary in Western descriptions and explanations of human experience, and consequently accounts couched in terms of the latter risk not being taken seriously.[40] In many ways, Civil-War Britain resembled parts of the modern world, where, as Boyden observed, the 'congruence of the human, natural and spiritual worlds are pivotal to the experience of suffering'.[41] For example, Imogen Peck has demonstrated how several women who lost their husbands fighting in the Civil Wars narrated their deaths in language of Providence. This was reflective of the tendency in early modern Britain to view worldly events as part of

[37] Joseph Lister, *The Autobiography of Joseph Lister of Bradford in Yorkshire*. Thomas Wright (ed), (London: John Russell Smith, 1842), pp. 7–8.

[38] Anne Laurence, 'Women's Work and the English Civil War', *History Today* 42, 1992, 20.

[39] Bracken, *Trauma*, pp. 6–7; Summerfield, 'Childhood, War, Refugeedom and 'Trauma'', p. 422.

[40] Ibid.

[41] Boyden, 'Children Under Fire', p. 13.

a God-given plan, which had widespread appeal in both traditional and more zealous contemporary religious cultures.[42]

Whilst there was much about the religious culture of Civil-War society that was extensive and shared, it is important to note the plurality of ways in which women and children engaged with religion in order to draw comfort. The options available to them were sometimes linked to considerations of social background, age and gender, and not all had uniformly positive side-effects. Ann Hughes noted that women were perhaps particularly affected by the loss of rituals that accompanied Parliament's attempts to reform the national church, as many of these were linked to crucial family events such as birth and marriage. Women such as Lady Isabella Twysden, a royalist sympathizer, clung to the old ways and continued to have her children baptized according to the traditional forms. Elsewhere, Anne Sadleir maintained a private chapel at Stanton Lordship, Hertfordshire, where worship persisted according to the Anglican liturgy banned by Parliament.[43] Maintaining old customs in the religious freedom afforded by a private chapel was not a luxury that extended beyond the elite. However, other avenues of religious expression were perhaps more readily available to the lower orders. As old forms of worship were swept away, new religious movements emerged as a result of the wars—spurred on by the commitment of Parliament's army to liberty of conscience—in which women played a prominent role.[44] Radical sects such as the Quakers offered apparent freedom to women, even women from the lower orders, to preach and publish. That said, the impudence displayed by some women in openly speaking against perceived ungodly social superiors provoked outrage. Such women were punished according to traditional humiliating and gender-specific penalties, such as the servant Dorothy Waugh, who was made to stand in Carlisle marketplace wearing the scold's bridle.[45] The social opprobrium displayed towards radical religious women is likely to have put off many others from joining their ranks.

[42] Imogen Peck, 'The Great Unknown: The Negotiation and Narration of Death by English War Widows, 1647–1660', *Northern History* 53, 2016, 229–30.

[43] Hughes, *Gender and the English Revolution*, pp. 71–72.

[44] Ibid., p. 74.

[45] Ibid., p. 82.

Although women's agency should not be negated, the outlets for religious comfort and expression available to them were often influenced by their husbands.[46] The influence of parents was likely to have placed even greater restrictions on the outlets available to children. That said, one area where children were given considerable freedom for religious expression was prophecy, which flourished in the turbulence of the Civil Wars. The fifteen-year-old Sarah Wight, having taken the rather alarming action of confining herself to her bed and refusing food, began to issue revelations on the grace of God in 1647.[47] Wight's family were linked to radical London churches and her insights were recorded by the Congregational minister Henry Jessey.[48] However, it should not be presumed that Wight was simply exploited by the adults that surrounded her. As Elizabeth Foyster argued, although adults might seek to control children's utterances, these might be taken very seriously in instances where they were perceived as speaking God's word, though the children often had to accompany their words with dramatic behaviour to secure an audience.[49] In fact, it was the very weakness and passivity of children, especially females, which made their prophecies plausible, as this chimed with Biblical assertions such as those of the prophet Joel that 'your sons and your daughters shall prophesy, your old men shall dream dreams, your young men shall see visions. And also upon the servants and upon the handmaid in those days will I pour out my spirit'.[50] The millenarian fervour which surrounded the Civil Wars may have made such beliefs especially popular but Karen Wells has shown how many cultures often accord children a divine or otherworldly status. She argued that this is based on the fact that childhood and children have been conceptualized

[46] Ibid., p. 74.

[47] Ibid., p. 77; Henry Jessey, *The Exceeding Riches of Grace Advanced By the Spirit of Grace, in an Empty Nothing Creature,* viz., *Mris Sarah Wight* (London, 1647).

[48] Hughes, *Gender and the English Revolution*, p. 77.

[49] Elizabeth Foyster, 'Silent Witnesses? Children and the Breakdown of Domestic and Social Disorder in Early Modern England', in Anthony Fletcher and Stephen Hussey (ed), *Childhood in Question: Children, Parents and the State*, ed. (Manchester: Manchester University Press, 1999), p. 65.

[50] Hughes, *Gender and the English Revolution*, p. 76.

as a liminal space and liminal subjects respectively, and consequently children are perceived to not occupy full social personhood.[51] With this in mind, the sacred status occasioned by children's liminality seems to have benefitted both children and adults during the Civil Wars: it enabled children to express their fears, hopes and dreams for the world of extreme uncertainty that they grew up into, whilst at the same time their prophecies provided adults with the comfort that there was a divine purpose to the turbulence of the times.

Family and Community

The influence of husbands and parents over the religious behaviour of women and children during the Civil Wars leads neatly to a consideration of the role of the family in survival strategies. Summerfield discerned that 'human pain' resulting from conflict is often 'managed within the family and community'.[52] Women and children in the Civil Wars seem to have sought strength in their families. This is perhaps unsurprising, given that evidence has shown that many early modern families across Europe exhibited gentle, loving and caring relations, including in their attitudes towards children.[53] Robert Harley claimed to his elder brother Edward that 'my desire is only to be with you'.[54] Sir William Fairfax, a colonel in Parliament's army in Northern England, was certainly under the impression that his wife, Lady Frances, received much comfort in his letters. He wrote to her following the battle of Marston Moor on 2 July 1644 that 'I know when you hear of our great battle with Prince Rupert you will be very fearfull of me; therefore I write to satisfie thee that God has also, at this time, preserved me from any hurt atall [sic.]'.[55] Some women, perhaps especially those from the lower social orders who were illiterate and thus unable to receive reassuring letters, took the drastic

[51] Karen Wells, 'Making Young Subjects: Liminality and Violence', in Nancy Worth, Clare Dwyer and Tracey Skelton (eds), *Geographies of Children and Young People: Identities and Subjectivities* (Berlin: Springer, 2016), pp. 215–30.

[52] Summerfield, 'Childhood, War, Refugeedom and "Trauma"', p. 421.

[53] Diana Gittins, 'The Historical Construction of Childhood', in Mary Jane Kehily (ed), *An Introduction to Childhood Studies* (Oxford: Oxford University Press, 2009), p. 43.

[54] *Manuscripts of His Grace the Duke of Portland*, vol. III, p. 110.

[55] Clements Markham, *Life of Robert Fairfax of Steeton, Vice-Admiral, Alderman, and Member for York A.D. 1666–1725* (London: Macmillan, 1885), p. 19.

measure of seeking out their husbands when no news was forthcoming. For example, Anne Norman from Darnton in County Durham travelled around fifty miles to Northallerton to seek out her husband, who was a soldier in Parliament's service.[56] As Peck pointed out, women like Norman would have been easy targets for crime—or might have risked being taken for criminals themselves—whilst the chances of successfully locating their husbands were bleak.[57]

Furthermore, evidence from the Civil Wars seems to reflect modern research that has demonstrated that the response of children to stressful events is often shaped by their parents and family.[58] According to Edward Halsall, resident with the countess of Derby throughout her defence of Lathom House, the countess's children, 'though truly apprehensive of the enemy's malice… were never startled by any appearance of danger'.[59] On one occasion, a missile burst into the dining-room during dinner. Allegedly, the girls 'scarcely changed colour'. Their mother gave them a look of approval and they continued their meal.[60] It need not be pointed out that these accounts were written to demonstrate the bravery of the royalist defence, though it may be speculated that the girls' strength in adversity was aided by the example of their formidable mother. At the very least, this example reveals that contemporary society had its own construction of the behavioural norms of each family member and, as in some parts of the modern world, containment of emotion and adaptation to circumstances were viewed as signs of maturity.[61] Women in the Civil Wars undoubtedly understood the value of publicly constraining their emotions. Andrew Hopper has highlighted how Katherine, Lady Brooke, painted herself as 'the stoic and patient puritan widow, who put suffering in the cause before her personal interests' in a petition to the House of Lords designed to remind them of the House of Commons' pledge to provide for her son Fulke. He was the posthumous son of

[56] Peck, 'The Great Unknown', p. 232.

[57] Ibid., p. 232.

[58] Summerfield, 'Childhood, War, Refugeedom and "Trauma"', p. 420; Andrea Doyle and Staci Perlman, 'Trauma Experienced in Adolescence', in Lisa Lopez Levers (ed), *Trauma Counselling: Theories and Interventions* (New York: Springer, 2012), p. 151.

[59] Halsall, 'Journal of the Siege of Lathom House', p. 515.

[60] Guizot de Witt, *The Lady of Latham; Being the Life and Original Letters of Charlotte de la Trémoille, Countess of Derby* (London: Smith, Elder & Co., 1869), p. 93.

[61] Summerfield, 'Childhood, War, Refugeedom and "Trauma"', p. 424.

the prominent parliamentarian Lord Brooke, who had been shot whilst besieging Lichfield in 1643.[62]

The lack of a public expression of emotion by some women and children in the Civil Wars should not detract from the impact of the loss of a loved one. Evidence from the Civil Wars perhaps reinforces research that suggests that parental absence or death might result in observed behavioural changes.[63] The thirteen-year-old Princess Elizabeth was inconsolable at the execution of her father Charles I, and said to have never fully recovered from her grief and shock. Sir Theodore Mayerne, the royal physician, commented that the princess 'fell into a great sorrow, whereby all other ailments from which she suffered were increased'. She died of a stomach tumour at Carisbrooke Castle on Isle of Wight in September 1650.[64] Physical illness is known to result in modern adolescents as a result of upsetting experiences.[65] That said, Elizabeth's track record of poor health may have played a more important role in her demise than royalist propagandists, keen to make political capital out of the unfortunate princess, were prepared to acknowledge.[66] When Lady Mary Verney returned to her family home in 1647, she discovered that her son had been spoilt rotten and his education neglected due to his father's exile in France, whilst her husband's sisters (whose own father had died at Edgehill) had become very insolent.[67] These youngsters may have been what is now described as 'acting out' because of painful experiences, although they may have—as Christopher Durston argued—simply have been relishing the freedom that the war afforded them through the absence of parents.[68] The insolence perceived by Mary may have been

[62] Andrew Hopper, '"To Condole with Me on the Commonwealth's Loss": The Widows and Orphans of Parliament's Military Commanders', in *Battle-Scarred*, ed. Appleby and Hopper, p. 195.

[63] Doyle and Perlman, 'Trauma Experienced in Adolescence', pp. 147, 150.

[64] Christopher Durston, *The Family in the English Revolution* (Oxford: Blackwell, 1989), p. 129.

[65] Doyle and Perlman, 'Trauma Experienced in Adolescence', p. 150.

[66] Thomas Herbert, *Memoirs of the Two Last Years of the Reign of Charles I by Sir Thomas Herbert, Groom to the Chambers to His Majesty* (London: G. and W. Nicol, 1813), pp. 178–79.

[67] Durston, *The Family*, pp. 128–29.

[68] Doyle and Perlman, 'Trauma Experienced in Adolescence', p. 147; Durston, *The Family*, p. 131.

as reflective of her own emotional disruption at having been forced to abandon her children.

Although developmental psychology has often stressed a safe, stable family environment as vital to children's wellbeing and normal development, several modern studies suggest that some children may be better able to accommodate dissonance and change than adults, though the long-term ramifications are not always clear.[69] Indeed there are many examples from the modern world where in situations of adversity, Children have had 'considerable positive impact on the psychological and emotional worlds of adults' and even become the carers of incapacitated adults or younger siblings.[70] Instances from the Civil Wars seem to reflect this phenomenon. For example, Thomas Spencer advised Lady Brooke to seek solace in her children.[71] Jonathan Priestley, admittedly writing from the perspective of hindsight as an adult, seemed to think that the death of his elder brother Sam had hit his mother especially hard in comparison to himself. Sam had died from fever contracted whilst rescuing a wounded comrade in Parliament's service when Jonathan was around nine to ten years old.[72]

In addition to challenging assumptions surrounding the roles performed by different family members in adverse situations, modern research has also questioned the necessity of a family in children's development at all and instead pointed to the importance of peers, school and neighbourhood networks in influencing behaviour.[73] In fact, community and wider social networks may be as important as 'the positive effects of family attachment' in helping people to adapt to difficult circumstances.[74] Jonathan noted with pride how 'Divers soldiers… some of them unknown to us' visited Sam in his last sickness, and the 'many friends' and 'neighbours about us' that joined the Priestley family at Sam's grave, inferring that he had found this neighbourly support helpful.[75] The prominence of

[69] Boyden, 'Children Under Fire', pp. 3, 15.

[70] Ibid., p. 15.

[71] Hopper, 'Widows and Orphans of Parliament's Military Commanders', p. 195.

[72] Charles Jackson, ed., *Memoirs of the Priestley Family* (Durham: Surtees Society, 1886), p. 27.

[73] Boyden, 'Children Under Fire', p. 10.

[74] Summerfield, 'Childhood, War, Refugeedom and "Trauma"', p. 421.

[75] Jackson, *Memoirs*, p. 27.

Lord Brooke to the parliamentarian cause meant that the parliamentarian elite rallied around Katherine and she received 'widespread recognition of her husband's sacrifice'.[76] She received many letters of condolence, including from one minister who presented her with a copy of verses that had been penned by her late husband.[77] The widows of the common soldiery may have received less individual public attention from the political establishment but support from their local communities appears to have been no less important in alleviating the effects of their loss. Jane verch Richard of Chirk in Denbighshire had been widowed when her husband was shot at Oswestry by royalist soldiers from Chirk Castle. When petitioning the Denbighshire Quarter Sessions for a war widow's pension, she paid testament to the community support she had received in informing the Justice of the Peace that she and her son had been 'left destitute of any meanes to mantayne themselues but what she hath of god & good people'.[78] Community support was particularly active in an age where few nuclear families could afford to be financially independent and notions of the virtues of 'good neighbourliness' governed 'a degree of normative consensus as to the nature of proper behaviour between neighbours'.[79]

Political Engagement

Faced with the death of a beloved relative, many women and children seem to have fortified themselves by asserting that the relative had not died in vain. William Fairfax, in a cruel twist of fate, was mortally wounded at Montgomery Castle two months after reassuring his wife that he had been unhurt at Marston Moor. According to the parliamentarian polemicist John Vicars, Lady Frances told her friends 'That shee greived not that hee dyed in this Cause, but that hee dyed so soon to doe no more for it'.[80] Vicars's account may need to be taken with a pinch of

[76] Hopper, 'Widows and Orphans of Parliament's Military Commanders', p. 196.

[77] Ibid., p. 195.

[78] National Library of Wales, Chirk Castle MS B8a/14 (petition of Jane verch Richard, 11 April 1648).

[79] Keith Wrightson, *English Society 1580–1680* (London: Hutchinson, 1982), pp. 51–57.

[80] John Vicars, *Magnalia Dei Anglicana. or, Englands Parliamentary Chronicle* (London: 1646), p. 34.

salt, but such sentiments were echoed elsewhere. Lady Elizabeth Capel's husband, Lord Arthur, had been captured following the royalist surrender of Colchester in August 1648. He was subsequently tried by Parliament and condemned to death. Throughout the trial, Arthur insisted that he had surrendered upon quarter and thus could not be proceeded against, a claim which was refuted by the parliamentarian commander-in-chief Thomas, Lord Fairfax. Elizabeth staunchly defended her husband's position, refusing to acknowledge the legitimacy of the court that tried him and claiming that his sentence was 'contrary to the knowne lawes of the land [and] the Priviledges of the Peeres of this Realme'.[81] Amongst the young, Jonathan Priestley asserted that his brother Sam's death was 'an act of compassion to the enemy'.[82]

Perhaps it should not be considered unusual that children in the Civil Wars responded to the loss and disruptions caused by the conflict by identifying with the political causes being fought over. Summerfield has observed that, in modern times, 'from El Salvador to Palestine to South Africa—children have actively identified themselves with social and political causes at stake'. He argued that such children should be regarded as 'Neither dupes nor straightforward victims' but their political engagement should be viewed in the context of their strength and ingenuity.[83] Political engagement amongst children during the Civil Wars was not merely confined to literate elites such as Priestley. In Exeter in January 1643, William Hutchenson, a canon of the cathedral, was 'abused and hooted at by the boys' as he was hauled through the streets as a prisoner by parliamentarian soldiers.[84] In Salisbury, a boy was imprisoned for allegedly saying that he would kill the king if he came to the city.[85] Such examples highlight the sometimes unedifying and dangerous side-effects of children's political engagement.

Despite the seemingly spontaneous nature of these political outbursts, the political creeds assumed by children to adapt to the environment

[81] Stewart Beale, 'War Widows and Revenge in Restoration England', *The Seventeenth Century* 33.2, 2018, 200–201.

[82] Jackson, *Memoirs*, p. 27.

[83] Summerfield, 'Childhood, War, Refugeedom and "Trauma"', p. 425.

[84] Mark Stoyle, *Locality and Loyalty: Popular Allegiance in Devon During the English Civil War* (Exeter: Exeter University Press, 1994), p. 101.

[85] *Mercurius Aulicus* 7 (12–18 February 1643), [2]–[3].

surrounding them were perhaps particularly susceptible to the influence of adults. Anne Bodvile petitioned Parliament that her children were being educated in 'opinions of averseness to the Parliament' by her mother-in-law. Her husband, the royalist colonel John Bodvile of Anglesey, had taken them away from her after they had fallen out. The House of Lords responded by ordering the three children to be placed in the care of their maternal grandfather, Sir William Russell.[86] The Bodvile case reveals that contemporaries did not consider it unusual for children to develop political opinions, although this might cause anxieties amongst adults. The disruptive consequences for these children of invoking such anxieties (almost certainly as a pretence to cover marital squabbling) need not be reiterated.

The rather unhealthier consequences of political engagement may be discerned for women too, especially amongst those women who drew strength from the perceived righteousness of their deceased husband's cause. Andrea Button examined the network of women in Southwest England who formed a 'pressure group' at the Restoration by petitioning Charles II to exempt former members of the Cromwellian judiciary from the General Pardon.[87] Their prime target was John Glynne, one of the judges who had condemned their husbands to death for their part in a royalist uprising during the Protectorate in 1655 and who had been deaf to the women's pleas for mercy at the time.[88] By exempting Glynne and his colleagues from the General Pardon, the women sought to bring them to justice for 'murdering' their husbands and moreover, the women demanded compensation out of what would be the confiscated estates of the condemned men.[89] Similarly, Stewart Beale has analyzed petitions submitted to the House of Lords during the first few months of the Restoration from gentry and aristocratic war widows, whose husbands had been tried and executed for treason during the 1640s and 1650s for their perceived loyalty to the royalist cause. Like the Southwestern pressure group, these women too demanded that their husbands' judges be excluded from the General Pardon and that compensation should be

[86] Durston, *The Family*, p. 126.

[87] Andrea Button, 'Royalist Women Petitioners in South-West England, 1655–62', *The Seventeenth Century* 15, 2000, 55.

[88] Ibid., p. 56.

[89] Ibid., p. 57.

awarded to them out of the estates of the men whom they wished to see condemned.[90]

Whilst this burning sense of injustice may have sustained the widows throughout the years of the Interregnum, it also spurred them on to a vindictive and perhaps self-destructive campaign for revenge. Mary Hewitt, the second wife of the royalist minister and conspirator Doctor John Hewitt, openly spoke of her 'unspeakable griefe' that resulted from her husband's execution in 1658; Elizabeth Burley, whose husband Captain John Burley had incited a royalist uprising on the Isle of Wight in 1647 and subsequently sentenced to death, alluded to her 'miserable & distressed condicon'.[91] Such rhetoric was, as Beale pointed out, designed to 'evoke feelings of sympathy within the addressee' and the petitioners cleverly drew on standardized tropes of female petitioning and royalist martyrology to fashion themselves as objects of pity.[92] However, these campaigns failed—with an effect on these women which can only be guessed at. Glynne not only survived but was created a serjeant-at-law by Charles, and most of the petitions submitted to the Lords were overlooked.[93] Judicial revenge was also largely a privilege reserved for the elite, though the widows of royalist conspirators who had been innkeepers and clothiers were part of the Southwestern 'pressure group'.[94]

In contrast to the women who assumed their husbands' political identity, others actively distanced themselves from their spouses' loyalty if their survival depended upon it. During the Civil Wars, Parliament confiscated royalists' estates, though these could be regained upon payment of a fine. It fell to many widows to negotiate the value of this fine with Parliament's 'Committee for Compounding'[95] Joan Heming of Poxwell in Dorset declared that her 'affections have always been very real to the Parliament and was very sollicitious w[i]th her said husband to bee like affected' in

[90] Stewart Beale, 'War Widows and Revenge in Restoration England', *The Seventeenth Century* 33, 2018, 195–217.

[91] Ibid., pp. 199, 203.

[92] Ibid., pp. 199–200.

[93] Button, 'Royalist Women Petitioners', p. 57; Beale, 'War Widows and Revenge', p. 210.

[94] Ibid., p. 197; Button, 'Royalist Women Petitioners', p. 56.

[95] Hannah Worthen, 'Supplicants and Guardians: The Petitions of Royalist Widows During the Civil Wars and Interregnum, 1642–1660', *Women's History Review* 26, 2017, 529.

an attempt to keep the cost of her fine down.[96] Others asserted their political ignorance. Mary Robinson of Branston, Lincolnshire, claimed to be 'ignorant of the cause' why her estate had been confiscated, though she later admitted to having sent her son to fight for the king furnished with a horse.[97] Claiming political ignorance was an easy survival tactic in a society which, despite widespread evidence for women's engagement, often exhibited a 'fundamental unease about women who were overtly influential in public life'.[98]

Poverty and Employment

The negotiation over estates is a reminder that the economic ramifications of war are often missing from studies of combat trauma. As Summerfield put it 'It may be somewhat arbitrary to talk of the trauma of war but not the trauma of poverty'.[99] Modern research has shown that a significant proportion of children who do suffer serious or prolonged psychological or emotional distress have been exposed not to dramatic circumstances but insidious hardships and deprivations, including poverty.[100] The Civil Wars resulted in significant property damage, trade slumps, agricultural decay, unemployment and inflation.[101] The population was subjected to unprecedented levels of taxation and (as we have seen) property confiscation.[102] Local societies were expected to billet soldiers, often without compensation, and were frequently in danger from plundering troops.[103] Mary Darrow of Down Hetherley in Gloucestershire was a widow who petitioned the parliamentarian governor of Gloucester, Edward Massie. She was 'much in debt... by reason of her great losse that in this distracted time she hath susteind' and could not pay 'the heavie taxes' that she was charged with. It was not only she herself who was forced to live with

[96] Ibid., p. 533.

[97] Ibid., p. 537.

[98] Hughes, *Gender and the English Revolution*, p. 49.

[99] Summerfield, 'Childhood, War, Refugeedom and "Trauma"', p. 418.

[100] Boyden, 'Children Under Fire', p. 20.

[101] Gentles, *English Revolution*, pp. 439–44.

[102] Ibid., pp. 444–45.

[103] Ibid., pp.445–49.

such financial straits but also her 'manie small Children'.[104] The loss of a husband/father deprived families of the principal breadwinner and might result in serious consequences. In Halstead, Essex, Margaret Johnson claimed that the death of her husband Abel in service in Ireland left her and her 'two small and sickly children' in 'a deplorable sad Condicion'.[105]

Of course, the language of poverty and distress were common tropes in the petitioning genre and perhaps this should be viewed more as testament to women's resourcefulness in mitigating the misfortunes of war than a reflection of their true situation and feelings.[106] David Appleby demonstrated in his study of maimed soldiers and war widows from Essex who petitioned their local courts of quarter sessions for financial relief that women employed more demonstrative language than their male counterparts and were better at presenting themselves as victims of war.[107] In a similar study, Andrew Hopper noted that even poor widows were more forthright than soldiers in quoting legal and moral precedent to the presiding justices, though this tendency was more noticeable amongst the widows of commanders. The latter were ready to voice feelings of grievance and entitlement because the targets of their petitions were of the same social status and often acquaintances of their deceased husbands.[108]

Lady Katherine Byron was the widow of Sir Thomas Byron, who had been lieutenant-colonel of the regiment commanded by Charles II (then Prince of Wales) himself. At the Restoration, Katherine did not hold back in informing the king that £700 lent by her husband to cover expenses in the regiment had not been repaid and reminded Charles that 'in consideration of her husbands former services your Father promised your Petitioner a Pencion'. She protested that she had been

> severall times plunderd, sequestred and endured long and cruell imprison[en]ts… being utterly Ruined of her fortune and forced to plead for her life… by the losse of her deare Husband and her other sufferings is

[104] The National Archives, SP 28/228/III, fol. 533 (petition of Mary Darrow, undated).

[105] Essex Record Office, Q/SBa2/84 (petition of Margaret Johnson, 1653).

[106] Worthen, 'Supplicants and Guardians', p. 532.

[107] David Appleby, 'Unnecessary Persons? Maimed Soldiers and War Widows in Essex, 1642–1662', *Essex Archaeology and History* 32, 2001, 213.

[108] Hopper, 'Widows and Orphans of Parliament's Military Commanders', p. 204.

> reduced to such extreamity that without yo[u]r Princely Compassion she is not longer able to support herselfe and Children.[109]

That the wife of a knight of the realm (and one who could afford to lend £700 at that) claimed poverty and suffering on behalf of herself and children may raise a few eyebrows. Yet, Boyden and Cooper argued that 'subjective' perceptions of life satisfaction often do not correlate in a straightforward way with 'objective' assessments of someone's material circumstances and 'relative poverty commonly has far more deleterious effect on psychological, emotional and social wellbeing than does absolute poverty'. This reflects the fact that 'material lack is perceived as far more debilitating when associated with stigma, social exclusion and denigration'.[110]

For poorer widows, remarriage often provided a way to navigate themselves and their families out of poverty. Many women lost husbands not only to the fighting but also to diseases such as plague brought by troops moving into new areas, but Paul Slack discovered that bereaved spouses were often quick to remarry.[111] Moreover, poorer women and children who sought to work their way out of poverty were paradoxically better placed than their social superiors. The resourcefulness gained by the former in the 'economy of makeshifts' placed them at an advantage in comparison to their more elevated counterparts, who lacked experience in paid employment and were likely to have found the prospect of this humiliating. Johan Illery informed the Devon justices that she had turned to 'spynning & carding' to eke out a living after her husband had been hanged for his allegiance to Parliament by Lord Paulet, the royalist victor at the siege of Hemyock Castle in 1644.[112] In the West Riding of Yorkshire, war widows were paid pensions only until their children were

[109] The National Archives, SP SP 29/14 fol. 71 (petition of Katherine Byron, 5 September 1660).

[110] Cooper and Boyden, 'Questioning the Power of Resilience', p. 8.

[111] Paul Slack, *The Impact of Plague in Tudor and Stuart England* (London: Routledge, 1985), p. 186.

[112] Devon Heritage Centre, QS Bundles, Box 51 (petition of Johan Illery, *c.* 1645–1646).

seven years old, as this was the age that the children could be bound for a parish apprenticeship and thus able to provide for themselves.[113]

To the modern mind, the concept of children working to provide for their families may seem shocking. Childhood is seen as a time that should be 'free of social and economic responsibility, and marked by learning and play' but this view rests on certain assumptions about children's needs and competencies and about the impact of environmental stressors on their development and wellbeing'.[114] Even less-privileged children in the Civil Wars still found time to play. According to the royalist newsbook *Mercurius Aulicus*, boys in Southampton organized themselves into 'Roundheads' and 'Cavaliers' and staged mock battles until allegedly their riotous behaviour brought them into trouble with the town government.[115] The diarist John Syms recorded a similar incident occurred in Plymouth on 27 March 1644, when the sermon he was attending in church was interrupted by the sound of children coming from outside crying 'Arme, Arme'! The men ran outside with swords drawn before realizing the cause of the commotion.[116] In fact, such violently themed play has been shown to be cathartic in contemporary societies, including many war zones, where this can be a useful way for children 'to achieve some mastery of an unstable environment'.[117] Nevertheless, as I have shown elsewhere, children in the seventeenth-century were expected to work and those who lived through the Civil Wars took on a number of jobs in the armies, which they performed with competence and sometimes even pride.[118]

[113] West Yorkshire History Centre, QS10/2, fol. 261 (West Riding of Yorkshire Quarter Sessions Order Book, April 1647 to August 1649); Steve Hindle, *On the Parish? The Micro-politics of Poor Relief in Rural England c. 1150–1750* (Oxford: Clarendon Press, 2004), p. 196.

[114] Boyden, 'Children Under Fire', p. 4.

[115] *Mercurius Aulicus* 16 (14–20 April 1644), 940. I am very grateful to Mark Stoyle for this reference.

[116] British Library, Additional MS 35297, (John Syms's day book, 1642–9). I am likewise grateful to Mark Stoyle for this reference.

[117] Rachel Rosen, 'Children's Violently Themed Play and Adult Imaginaries of Childhood: A Bakhtinian Analysis', *International Journal of Early Childhood* 47, 2015, 236–37; Summerfield, 'Childhood, War, Refugeedom and "Trauma"', p. 429.

[118] Pells, 'Children, Childhood and Armies During the British Civil Wars'.

Although children are often perceived to have fewer survival strategies available to them than adults, the reverse is often true 'because societies tend to be less prescriptive about children's tasks and roles'. Adults frequently pay little attention to children, making 'it possible for them to undertake tasks that adults are barred from, such as foraging and scavenging in areas controlled by security forces'.[119] It is noticeable that many boys in the Civil Wars acted as spies or scouts and played an important role in foraging.[120] Modern research has demonstrated that child-rearing which emphasizes independence and gives children a sense of responsibility, including income-generation, promotes well-being, self-efficacy and social skills'.[121] Indeed, the impact on children whose livelihood was taken away from them as a result of the Civil Wars is worth considering. When parliamentarian soldiers and their local supporters defaced Exeter Cathedral and plundered the Cathedral Close, they marched past crestfallen choristers having just ripped out the Cathedral organ pipes, jeering 'Boys, we have spoilt your trade, you must go sing hot pudding pies!'[122]

A similar question might be asked of the women. Many women found employment as a result of the Civil Wars. For example, amongst the payments made by Parliament's New Model Army were disbursements to Mary Roberts 'a female scout', Anne Meacock and Elizabeth Alkin for medical provision, and Susan Bowen for the rather enigmatic 'special service'.[123] As Barton Hacker speculated, the freedom enjoyed by women employed in the military may have been 'real enough in contrast to the constraints of rural poverty or urban slum from which they had come and to which, without the army, they had no choice but to return'.[124] Indeed, one woman who had been a camp follower in the Thirty Years' War, the European conflict contemporaneous with the Civil Wars, apparently bemoaned the end of the fighting by saying 'I was born in war, I have no home, no country and no friends; war is all my wealth and

[119] Boyden, 'Children Under Fire', p. 16.

[120] Pells, 'Children, Childhood and Armies During the British Civil Wars'.

[121] Boyden, 'Children Under Fire', p. 17.

[122] Stoyle, *Locality and Loyalty*, pp. 106–107.

[123] E. Kitson and E. Kitson Clark, 'Some Civil War Accounts, 1647–1650', *The Thoresby Society Publications* XI, Miscellanea IV (1904), 164, 172, 198, 200.

[124] Barton Hacker, 'Women and Military Institutions in Early Modern Europe: A Reconnaissance', *Signs* 6, 1981, 663.

now whither shall I go?'.[125] The fate of veteran soldiers after demobilization has been a recent subject of study, but what was the impact of the disbandment of the armies on the women who followed them?[126]

Conclusion

In moving away from the modern and medical language of trauma, it has not been my intention to downplay the suffering that women and children in the British Civil Wars may have experienced or to deny the possibility that the conflict resulted in psychological disorders for some. However, it was my aim to demonstrate that women and children in the Civil Wars had to adapt to the militarisation of the world around them and as historians, we should pay attention to the individual ways in which they mitigated the influence of violence and disruption.[127] As Summerfield concluded, whilst the concept of trauma may continue to be fashionable in some quarters, 'it is the social, cultural, and economic rebuilding of worlds shattered by war (including valued institutions such as schools), allied to urgent issues of equity and justice, which will determine the future wellbeing of several million child survivors worldwide'.[128]

By studying the social, cultural, economic and political frameworks to which those in the past turned to reimpose meaning and order on their disrupted lives, we can gain a better understanding of the nuances of how these frameworks might operate in different contexts. Furthermore, a study of women and children specifically brings a different perspective to the scholarship on the psychological impact of the Civil Wars. It highlights how the survival strategies available to contemporaries often varied according to gender and age, as well as the socio-economic environment and political or cultural circumstances. At the same time, by taking advantage of the long view afforded by the benefits of hindsight, an historical study can draw attention to some of the ways in which different approaches may have been positive sources of strength in the

[125] Ibid., pp. 654.

[126] See for example, Appleby, 'Veteran Politics in Restoration England', pp. 323–42.

[127] Summerfield, 'Childhood, War, Refugeedom and "Trauma"', pp. 419, 421.

[128] Derek Summerfield, 'Protecting Children from Armed Conflict. Children Affected by War Must Not Be Stigmatised as Permanently Damaged', *BMJ Clinical Research* 317, 1998, 1249.

immediate aftermath of a disruptive event but have unforeseen negative long-term effects. This can act as a reminder of the shortcomings of resilience discourse and the unhelpfulness of value judgements about 'overcoming adversity'.

Nevertheless, as Boyden explained, arguing the individuals may be resourceful in difficult situations does not imply that they should be expected to tolerate hardship or that a violent environment is necessarily a propitious one but it does 'bring into question the inevitability of catastrophic effects' and enables us to acknowledge the importance of an individual's own efforts towards their survival.[129] The themes raised in this chapter would all benefit from further challenge, discussion and development. However, what I have shown is that the women and children who lived through the Civil Wars were far from helpless victims, but navigated the violence, disruption, and human tragedy that this conflict entailed with courage and ingenuity.

Bibliography

Appleby, David, 'Unnecessary Persons? Maimed Soldiers and War Widows in Essex, 1642–1662', *Essex Archaeology and History* 32, 2001, 209–21.

Appleby, David, 'Veteran Politics in Restoration England, 1660–1670,' *The Seventeenth Century* 28, 2013, 323–42.

Beale, Stewart, 'War Widows and Revenge in Restoration England', *The Seventeenth Century* 33, 2018, 195–217.

Bottrell, Dorothy, 'Responsibilised Resilience? Reworking Neoliberal Social Policy Texts', *M/C Journal* 16, 2013, https://doi.org/10.5204/mcj.708

Boyden, Jo, 'Children Under Fire: Challenging Assumptions About Children's Resilience', *Children, Youth and Environments* 13, 2003, 1–29.

Bracken, Patrick, *Trauma: Culture, Meaning and Philosophy* (London: Whurr, 2002).

British Library, Additional MS 35297 (John Syms's day book, 1642–9).

Button, Andrea, 'Royalist Women Petitioners in South-West England, 1655–62', *The Seventeenth Century* 15, 2000, 53–66.

Cooper, Elizabeth and Jo Boyden, 'Questioning the Power of Resilience: Are Children Up to the Task of Disrupting the Transmission of Poverty?' *Chronic Poverty Research Centre Working Paper* 73, 2007, 1–20 https://doi.org/10.2139/ssrn.1753009

[129] Boyden, 'Children Under Fire', pp. 15–16.

Devon Heritage Centre, QS Bundles, Box 51 (petition of Johan Illery, *c.* 1645–6).

de Witt, Guizot, *The Lady of Latham; Being the Life and Original Letters of Charlotte de la Trémoille, Countess of Derby* (London: Smith, Elder & Co., 1869).

Dowdney, Linda, 'Trauma, Resilience and Cultural Hearing: How Do We Move Forward?' *Child Soldiers International Psychosocial Paper*, 2007, 2–3.

Doyle, Andrea and Staci Perlman, 'Trauma Experienced in Adolescence', in Lisa Lopez Levers (ed), *Trauma Counselling: Theories and Interventions* (New York: Springer, 2012), pp. 146–60.

Durston, Christopher, *The Family in the English Revolution* (Oxford: Blackwell, 1989).

Essex Record Office, Q/SBa2/84 (petition of Margaret Johnson, 1653).

Halsall, Edward, 'A Journal of the Siege of Lathom House', in Julis Hutchinson (ed), *Memoirs of the Life of Colonel Hutchinson* (London: Henry G. Bohn, 1848), pp. 491–518

Foyster, Elizabeth, 'Silent Witnesses? Children and the Breakdown of Domestic and Social Disorder in Early Modern England', in Anthony Fletcher and Stephen Hussey (eds), *Childhood in Question: Children, Parents and the State* (Manchester: Manchester University Press, 1999), pp. 57–73.

Garrett, Paul, 'Questioning Tales of "Ordinary Magic": "Resilience" and Neo-Liberal Reasoning', *British Journal of Social Work* 46, 2016, 1909–25.

Gentles, Ian, *The English Revolution and the Wars in the Three Kingdoms, 1638–1652* (London: Pearson Education, 2007).

Gittins, Diana, 'The Historical Construction of Childhood', in Mary Jane Kehily (ed), *An Introduction to Childhood Studies* (Oxford: Oxford University Press, 2009), pp. 35–49.

Hacker, Barton, 'Women and Military Institutions in Early Modern Europe: A Reconnaissance', *Signs* 6, 1981, 643–71.

Herbert, Thomas, *Memoirs of the Two Last Years of the Reign of Charles I by Sir Thomas Herbert, Groom to the Chambers to His Majesty* (London: G. and W. Nicol, 1813).

Hindle, Steve, *On the Parish? The Micro-politics of Poor Relief in Rural England c. 1150–1750* (Oxford: Clarendon Press, 2004).

Hopper, Andrew, '"To Condole with Me on the Commonwealth's Loss": The Widows and Orphans of Parliament's Military Commanders', in David Appleby and Andrew Hopper (eds), *Battle-Scarred: Mortality, Medical Care and Military Welfare in the British Civil Wars* (Manchester: Manchester University Press, 2018), pp. 174–91.

Hughes, Ann, *Gender and the English Revolution* (Abingdon: Routledge, 2012).

Jackson, Charles (ed), *Memoirs of the Priestley Family* (Durham: Surtees Society, 1886).

Jessey, Henry, *The Exceeding Riches of Grace Advanced by the Spirit of Grace, in an Empty Nothing Creature, viz., Mris Sarah Wight* (London, 1647).

Kitson, E. and E. Kitson Clark, 'Some Civil War Accounts, 1647–1650', *The Thoresby Society Publications* XI, Miscellanea IV (1904), 137–235.

Laurence, Anne, 'Women's Work and the English Civil War', *History Today* 42, 1992, 20–25.

Lister, Joseph, *The Autobiography of Joseph Lister of Bradford in Yorkshire*, Thomas Wright (ed), (London: John Russell Smith, 1842).

Markham, Clements, *Life of Robert Fairfax of Steeton, Vice-Admiral, Alderman, and Member for York A.D. 1666–1725* (London: Macmillan, 1885).

Mercurius Aulicus 16 (14–20 April 1644).

Mercurius Aulicus 7 (12–18 February 1643).

National Library of Wales, Chirk Castle MS B8a/14 (petition of Jane verch Richard, 11 April 1648).

Peck, Imogen, 'The Great Unknown: The Negotiation and Narration of Death by English War Widows, 1647–1660', *Northern History* 53, 2016, 220–35.

Pells, Ismini, 'Children, Childhood and Armies During the British Civil Wars', forthcoming.

Pells, Ismini, 'Soliciting Sympathy: The Search for Psychological Trauma in Seventeenth-Century English Civil War Maimed Soldiers' Petitions', in Erin Peters and Cynthia Richards (eds), *Early Modern Trauma: Europe and the Atlantic World* (Lincoln, NE: University of Nebraska Press, 2021), pp. 129–50.

Peters, Erin, '"The Deep Staines These Wars Will Leave Behind": Psychological Wounds and Curative Methods in the English Civil Wars', in David Appleby and Andrew Hopper (eds), *Battle-Scarred: Mortality, Medical Care and Military Welfare in the British Civil Wars* (Manchester: Manchester University Press, 2018), pp. 156–73.

Peters, Erin, 'Trauma Narratives of the English Civil War', *Journal for Early Modern Cultural Studies* 16, 2016, 78–94.

Roberts, Stephen (ed), 'Surnames Beginning "H"', *The Cromwell Association Online Directory of Parliamentarian Army Officers* (2017), https://www.british-history.ac.uk/no-series/cromwell-army-officers/surnames-h, accessed 19 February 2018.

Rosen, Rachel, 'Children's Violently Themed Play and Adult Imaginaries of Childhood: A Bakhtinian Analysis', *International Journal of Early Childhood* 47, 2015, 235–50.

Slack, Paul, *The Impact of Plague in Tudor and Stuart England* (London: Routledge, 1985).

Stoyle, Mark, '"Give mee a Souldier's Coat": Female Cross-Dressing During the English Civil War', *History* 103, 2018, 5–26.

Stoyle, Mark, *Locality and Loyalty: Popular Allegiance in Devon During the English Civil War* (Exeter: Exeter University Press, 1994).

Summerfield, Derek, 'Childhood, War, Refugeedom and "Trauma": Three Core Questions for Mental Health Professionals', *Journal of Transcultural Psychiatry* 37, 2000, 417–33.

Summerfield, Derek, 'Protecting Children from Armed Conflict. Children Affected by War Must Not Be Stigmatised as Permanently Damaged', *BMJ Clinical Research* 317, 1998, 1549–50.

The Manuscripts of His Grace the Duke of Portland: Preserved at Welbeck Abbey (10 vols, London: H.M.S.O, 1891–1931).

The National Archives, SP 28/228/III, fol. 533 (petition of Mary Darrow, undated).

The National Archives, SP SP 29/14 fol. 71 (petition of Katherine Byron, 5 September 1660).

Ungar, Michael, 'Introduction: Resilience Across Cultures and Contexts', in Michael Ungar (ed), *Handbook for Working with Children and Youth: Pathways to Resilience Across Cultures and Contexts* (London: Sage, 2005), pp. xvix–xxix.

Vicars, John, *Magnalia Dei Anglicana. or, Englands Parliamentary Chronicle* (London, 1646).

Warburton, Eliot, *Memoirs of Prince Rupert and the Cavaliers* (London: Richard Bentley, 1849).

Wells, Karen, 'Making Young Subjects: Liminality and Violence', in Nancy Worth, Clare Dwyer and Tracey Skelton (eds), *Geographies of Children and Young People: Identities and Subjectivities* (Berlin: Springer, 2016), pp. 215–30.

West Yorkshire History Centre, QS10/2, fol. 261 (West Riding of Yorkshire Quarter Sessions Order Book, April 1647 to August 1649).

Worthen, Hannah, 'Supplicants and Guardians: The Petitions of Royalist Widows During the Civil Wars and Interregnum, 1642–1660', *Women's History Review* 26, 2017, 528–40.

Wrightson, Keith, *English Society 1580–1680* (London: Hutchinson, 1982).

Index

O. Rees et al. (eds.), *Combat Stress in Pre-modern Europe*, Mental Health in Historical Perspective,
https://doi.org/10.1007/978-3-031-09947-2

The manufacturer's authorised representative in the EU is Springer Nature Customer Service Centre GmbH, Europaplatz 3, 69115 Heidelberg, Germany. If you have any concerns regarding our products, please contact ProductSafety@springernature.com

Printed and bound by CPI Group (UK) Ltd, Croydon, CR0 4YY

30/09/2026

02225243-0002